To:
Captain Hight C. Warwick

AAFTTC 5th District

Miami Beach Fla.

With Compliments of
John Charles Long Jr.

ENDOTRACHEAL ANAESTHESIA

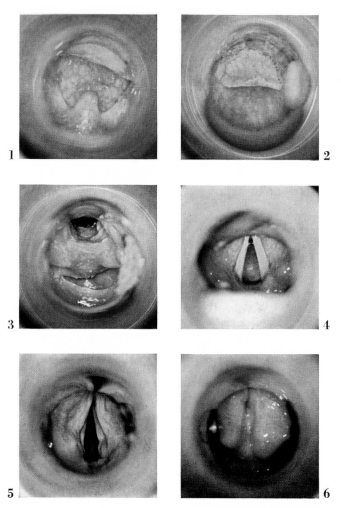

1. Tongue, posterior pharyngeal wall, fauces, and uvula as seen when the laryngoscope is inserted into the mouth. 2. The epiglottis exposed. 3. View of the posterior half of the glottis when the epiglottis has been partially lifted. 4. The glottis fully exposed. 5. A fully exposed and completely relaxed glottis. 6. A fully exposed glottis in spasm.

Endotracheal Anaesthesia

By

NOEL A. GILLESPIE

D.M., B.ch., M.A. (OXON.); D.A. (R.C.S. ENG.)

Research Associate and Resident in Anaesthesia
University of Wisconsin: State of Wisconsin
General Hospital

Sometime:

Senior Resident Anaesthetist, The London Hospital

Hon. Assistant Anaesthetist, The London Hospital

Hon. Assistant Instructor in Anaesthetics, London Hospital
Medical College and Dental School

Hon. Anaesthetist, The Connaught Hospital, Walthamstow

Anaesthetist to the Plastic Department, Princess Elizabeth of
York Hospital for Children, Shadwell

THE UNIVERSITY OF WISCONSIN PRESS

1941

FOREWORD

THE AUTHOR of this monograph has repeatedly and severally admonished the three undersigned musketeers to write a dissertation covering the subject of endotracheal anaesthesia. Although we had each agreed that such an effort was desirable, through busyness or more probably because of that personal inertia rarely but more honestly referred to as laziness, we have each postponed compliance with his courteous request.

It is fitting that the work has finally been accomplished by one who is younger and whose attitude is, for that reason and through varied experience, less biased than that of any of us. Certainly the meticulous care with which the historical aspects of the subject have been ferreted out could not have been equalled by us who are possessed neither of the time nor the patience for such a labor.

It is with confidence, therefore, that we commend to present and future anaesthetists this excellent treatise which we believe covers adequately to date the historical, theoretical, and practical aspects of endotracheal intubation as it applies to the administration of volatile and gaseous agents.

It is our sincere hope and belief that this little book will serve as a foundation upon which may be built improvements in principles and technique which will make endotracheal anaesthesia an even more useful aid than we have found it in the struggle to bring help to surgeons and comfort and safety to patients.

I. W. MAGILL
RALPH WATERS
ARTHUR GUEDEL

AUTHOR'S PREFACE

In the past decade the advantages of endotracheal anaesthesia have increasingly won recognition until now any specialist in anaesthesia is expected to possess both skill and experience in the use of this technique. Thus far, as the references and bibliography of this book show, anyone wishing to learn of the work previously done in this field had to consult so large a number of works in periodicals so widely scattered that he could only hope to do so if he had access to a well-stocked medical library, and could devote a considerable amount of time to reading. Having encountered this difficulty myself in the past, I have felt for some years that it would be of assistance to anaesthetists if the facts could be collected in one small volume. It is the function of this monograph to present the salient facts concisely, and to include a bibliography and references such that any reader sufficiently interested may be able readily to refer to the original sources.

I can only advance three excuses for my temerity in undertaking a task to which I feel myself to be inadequate. The first of these is that my present appointment has provided me with an opportunity and facilities probably unrivalled in the world, for which I am deeply grateful to the State of Wisconsin University Hospital. The second is that it has been my privilege to be associated with several colleagues who have made outstanding contributions to the subject, and that I hope to share with the reader the facts and opinions learned from them. The third is that I have had the opportunity of acquiring some experience at first hand in the management of the method. Whatever is worth while in this book has been inspired by my leaders and friends Ralph Waters, Ivan Magill, Arthur Guedel, and Michael Nosworthy. For its deficiencies, negligences, and ignorances I alone am responsible.

The "insufflation" technique is but rarely used nowadays. It has therefore been considered in an early chapter, the remainder of the book being concerned primarily with "inhalation" endotracheal anaesthesia. The form in which the references appear has been adopted partly because it is concise, and partly because, in the author's experience, the year, volume, and page are sufficient data to enable any article to be found without difficulty.

It is a pleasant duty to record my indebtedness and gratitude to many friends who have helped in the labor of compiling this book. I am beholden to my chief, Dr. R. M. Waters, to Dr. A. E. Guedel and Dr. W. H. Cassels, and to my colleagues of the Department of Anaesthesia of the Wisconsin General Hospital for reading the rough draft, for their helpful criticisms and suggestions, and for their encouragement. Dr. Paul H. Holinger of Chicago has kindly allowed me to reproduce his excellent color photographs to illustrate the steps involved in laryngoscopy, and I am most grateful for this courtesy. I am indebted to Dr. and Mrs. F. C. Jacobson and to Miss Elisabeth Miller for their skilful execution of the line drawings and diagrams. At the Wisconsin General Hospital Mr. J. G. Diebold of the photographic department and Mr. J. P. Dean of the radiological department have very kindly put their technical skill at my disposal in helping to produce the illustrations. Drs. P. J. Flagg, P. D. Woodbridge, and F. W. Clement have kindly given me permission to take or reproduce photographs of apparatus, and the staff of the University of Wisconsin Press has spared neither time nor trouble in helping to prepare this monograph for publication. Finally, I gratefully acknowledge the permission granted by the firms of A. Charles King Ltd. and Divided Airways Ltd. to reproduce illustrations of apparatus made by them and my indebtedness to Mr. Charles King and Mr. H. A. E. Talley personally for their help in this and many other matters.

The wider availability of endotracheal anaesthesia depends upon an increasing supply of medical men conversant with the facts and skilled by long experience in the technique of intubating the trachea. It is the author's hope that this monograph may thus enable more patients to reap the benefits accruing both to surgery and to anaesthesia from the exhibition of endotracheal methods.   N.A.G.

CONTENTS

LIST OF FIGURES

Fortiter in re: suaviter in modo

INTRODUCTION

"ENDOTRACHEAL" AND "INTRATRACHEAL" anaesthesia are the terms used to describe the administration of anaesthetic vapors directly into the trachea by means of a tube passed into it through the larynx from the mouth or nose. The former word is derived from the Greek adverb ἔνδον, which signifies "inside," and τραχεῖα, the feminine of the adjective τραχύς, which signifies "rough." The structure we now call the "trachea" was referred to by the ancients as τραχεῖα ἄρτηρια (the rough vessel), and even in the middle of the seventeenth century Robert Hook termed it *aspera arteria*.[1] The word "intratracheal" has resulted from the substitution of the Latin preposition *intra*, meaning "within," for its Greek counterpart. The terms are therefore synonymous, the first being probably the more correct inasmuch as it consistently derives from the language of source. Ever since this technique of anaesthesia has been in use the two terms have been equally current in the English-speaking countries, and their use has been adopted for the purpose by several Continental nations.

Endotracheal tubes may be passed into the trachea either through the mouth or through the nose. It seems logical to describe such anaesthetics as "orotracheal" and "nasotracheal" respectively. These words are derived from the Latin *os* (the mouth) and *nasus* (the nose). The Greek forms would be cumbersome as "stomotracheal" and "rhinotracheal," and might lead to confusion in this unlettered age! The term "orotracheal" has the sanction of precedent, having been used by Hill[2] before the Royal Society of Medicine in 1914.

"INHALATION" AND "INSUFFLATION"

A perusal of the literature shows that two different principles may be applied to the administration of an endotracheal anaes-

3

thetic. They have come to be known as "inhalation" and "insufflation." In endotracheal inhalation the patient both inhales and exhales through a wide-bore tube placed in the trachea. The anaesthetic vapor is supplied to this tube from a bag at atmospheric pressure. If the patient's own respiratory movements become deficient, alveolar exchange can be assisted by manual pressure upon the bag. In endotracheal insufflation the anaesthetic vapor is forced into the trachea by positive pressure through a narrow-bore tube whose end lies close to the bifurcation. The returning gases find their way out between the wall of this tube and that of the trachea. A constant partial distension of the lungs is maintained by the insufflation pressure used; if this pressure is raised sufficiently and the outflow is rapid enough, cessation of respiratory movements ensues.

A third principle has been used by some workers. It is really a variant of the inhalation technique, for it consists of using a wide-bore tube placed in the trachea as an airway for the patient's respirations, and, by means of a side-tube, injecting into it an appropriate quantity of the anaesthetic agent. Modern examples of this technique are Magill's "chloroform adaptor" [3] and Ayre's T-tube. [4]

The historical evolution of these different principles is outlined in Chapter I. Inhalation made its appearance first, to be temporarily eclipsed by insufflation during the period from 1909 to 1926. Then the tide turned again, until now inhalation has almost entirely superseded insufflation. This latter trend has, however, been gradual, and has been accelerated by factors other than the intrinsic value of either principle. Physiological respiration takes place in both directions through a wide-bore tube, and apnoea does not normally occur, although it may do so in response to alterations in the threshold of the respiratory centre to stimulus, or to variations in intensity of such stimuli. Inhalation, therefore, more closely resembles normal respiration than does insufflation. For this reason the insufflation principle has been dealt with in Chapter III, the rest of the book being concerned with inhalation endotracheal anaesthesia.

SCIENCE AND ART

The modern devotion to Science, which is exact, as opposed to Art, which is not exact, has one disastrous consequence when applied to the practice of medicine. The devotees of the "scientific" attitude are wont to seek "indications" and "contra-indications," and to apply them by rule of thumb to all patients who exhibit certain symptoms or signs. "Routine" should have no place in medicine, for all "indications" and "contra-indications" are relative rather than absolute. Each case is a problem in itself, and must be so considered. Of nothing is this more true than of endotracheal anaesthesia. Therefore in this book an attempt will be made to discuss the arguments for and against each detail of the method rather than to state "indications" and "contra-indications." Endotracheal anaesthesia is a valuable technique which has profoundly modified both the patient's safety and the surgeon's freedom of access and asepsis, and hence the anaesthetist's peace of mind. Some enthusiasts have therefore attempted to use it as a "routine" in all patients and for every variety of operation. Nevertheless its use necessitates a delicate operation, fraught with risks of trauma which vary inversely as the skill and experience of the intubator. Endotracheal anaesthesia should always be available to any patient who may benefit from it: it should never be used without good cause.

REFERENCES

1. HOOK, R. Phil. Trans. Roy. Soc. 1667. II. 539.
2. HILL, W. Proc. Roy. Soc. Med. (Anaes.) 1914. VII. 36.
3. *Vide:* Nosworthy, M. D. Theory and Practice of Anaesthesia. 1st ed. London, 1932. p. 137.
4. AYRE, P. Brit. Jour. Surg. 1937. XXV. 131.

I. THE HISTORY OF ENDOTRACHEAL ANAESTHESIA

INTUBATION OF THE TRACHEA for purposes of resuscitation is three centuries older than anaesthesia itself. In 1542 Vesalius[1] recorded the experiment of passing a reed into the *aspera arteria* of an animal whose thorax had been opened, and blowing into it intermittently. He found that this caused the lungs to expand, and the heart to recover its normal pulsation.*

Just over a century later Robert Hook[2] performed a similar experiment before the Royal Society of London. His own account of this "Noble Experiment," performed on October 24, 1667, is both illuminating and diverting:

I did heretofore give this Illustrious Society an account of an Experiment I formerly tryed of keeping a Dog alive after his Thorax was all display'd by the cutting away of the Ribs and Diaphragme; and after the Pericardium of the heart also was taken off . . . the Dog being kept alive by the Reciprocal blowing up of his Lungs with Bellowes, and they suffered to subside, for the space of an hour or more, after his Thorax had been so display'd, and his Aspera Arteria cut off just below the Epiglotis, and bound on upon the nose of the Bellows.

He found that when he ceased to inflate the lungs the dog developed convulsive motions. Then he joined a second pair of bellows to the first in order to provide a constant stream of air,

and pricking all the outer-coat of the Lungs with the slender point of a very sharp pen-knive, the second pair of Bellows was mov'd very quick, whereby the first pair was always kept very full and always blowing into the lungs; by which means the Lungs also were kept very full, and without any motion,

* He also noticed that if the lungs were allowed to remain collapsed, the pulsation of the heart and arteries became, "undosus, formicans, et vermicularis" (wave-like, ant-like, and worm-like). It is remarkable to find so good a description, at so early a date, of what we have since come to call "ventricular fibrillation."

6

there being a continual blast of air forc'd into the Lungs by the first pair of Bellows, supplying it as fast, as it could find its way quite through the Coat of the Lungs by the small holes pricked in it, as was said before. This being continued for a pretty while, the dog, as I expected, lay still as before, his eyes being all the time very quick, and his Heart beating very regularly: But, upon ceasing the Blast and suffering the Lungs to fall and lye still, the Dog would immediately fall into Dying Convulsive fits; but he as soon revived again by the renewing the fulness of his Lungs with the constant blast of fresh air.

He concludes:

So it was not the subsiding or movelesness of the Lungs that was the immediate cause of Death, or the stopping of the circulation of the Blood through the Lungs, but the want of a sufficient supply of fresh air.

Towards the close of the eighteenth century intubation of the trachea as a means of artificial respiration in cases of asphyxia or drowning became fairly common. It is evident, from the work of J. Leroy[3, 4] that the forcible insufflation of air into the trachea with bellows, which was then a current practice, often did more harm than good because it was not sufficiently realized that a sudden excess of pressure was dangerous and that there must be provision for expiration as well as inspiration. Moreover, Leroy showed by animal experiments that the production of pneumothorax from rupture of the alveoli was perfectly possible if the lungs were forcibly over-inflated. He therefore suggested that the handles of the bellows be provided with a safety stop-catch to prevent over-distension of the lungs. He also devised a primitive precursor of the modern laryngoscope intended to facilitate the introduction of a tube into the trachea. His work was investigated by Magendie,[5] who reported favorably on it to the Academie des Sciences. A great deal of work was done on resuscitation in the course of the nineteenth century, but it does not directly concern us.

It is perhaps appropriate that what is now the recognized technique of the physiologist for administering an anaesthetic over a long period of time should have originated with John Snow.[6] In or before 1858, when his book *On Chloroform and Other Anaesthetics* was published, he administered an endotracheal chloroform anaesthesia to a rabbit by performing tracheotomy and inserting into the trachea a wide-bore tube through which the animal breathed in and out of a bag filled with chloroform vapor.

In 1871 Friedrich Trendelenburg[7] used this method in man. He was seeking a solution to the problem of preventing the aspiration of blood into the lungs during operations upon the upper air passages; and he achieved this by performing a preliminary tracheotomy through the opening of which a wide-bore tube was passed into the trachea. This tube carried an inflatable cuff which made "watertight" contact with the tracheal wall; and it was connected by a length of rubber tubing to a funnel covered with gauze or flannel. Anaesthesia was maintained by dropping chloroform on the gauze. In spite of the mutilation inherent in the method it enjoyed a considerable vogue at the time.

Endotracheal anaesthesia, as we know it at the present day, was born in Glasgow in 1880. William MacEwen,[8] who wished to remove an extensive malignant growth from the base of a patient's tongue, was seeking a method that would permit of the smooth and continuous administration of the anaesthetic, and of the protection of the respiratory tract from the aspiration of blood. He had already carried out experiments on intubation of the trachea in the cadaver, and had concluded that the nasal route was unsuitable because the course of the nares in the normal subject inclines medially. Thus a tube passed through the right nostril crosses the middle line in the pharynx and tends to meet the left false cord, and vice versa (see Figure 27 on page 84). He found, however, that he could easily insert a metal tube into the trachea through the mouth by the sense of touch. Intubation was carried out several times upon the patient without anaesthesia in the preoperative period. When it was found that no undue disturbance was caused by the intubation, chloroform was administered through the tube, the laryngeal opening was packed off, and the operation was successfully performed. He recorded two other cases in which he used intubation successfully in the treatment of respiratory obstruction resulting from oedema of the glottis. He then attempted to use it again in a case similar to the first. The patient, who had been intubated before the induction of anaesthesia, requested that the tube be removed during induction and re-inserted later. The tube was removed and induction begun. The patient, however, struggled violently during the second stage of anaesthesia and died of cardiac failure before the operation could be started.

In 1893 Maydl,[9] professor of surgery in Prague, suggested "the intubation of the larynx to prevent the ingress of blood into the organs of respiration during operation." By then the classic work of O'Dwyer[10] on intubation in diphtheria was well known, and Maydl conceived the idea of adapting the technique of laryngeal intubation to the needs of anaesthesia for oto-rhino-laryngological operations. Since no operation can be adequately carried out if it must be interrupted periodically for the re-anaesthetization of the patient, it was not only necessary to find some method of preventing the aspiration of blood and operative debris into the respiratory tract, but also of resolving the constant conflict of access to the patient's face between surgeon and anesthetist. Maydl therefore devised a laryngeal tube, closely resembling that of O'Dwyer, which could be connected to the type of funnel used by Trendelenburg. When the intubation had been performed, the pharynx was tightly packed with gauze around the tube. Apparently this arrangement functioned satisfactorily in spite of the large amount of rebreathing which took place in the rubber tube connecting the laryngeal tube to the funnel. Eisenmenger,[11] who may have been familiar with the work of Trendelenburg, published a description of a tube which he had invented for use with Maydl's technique. It was a wide-bore semi-rigid tracheal tube carrying an inflatable cuff of the variety suggested by Trendelenburg (Figure 1).

George Bernard Shaw has wittily drawn attention[12] to the

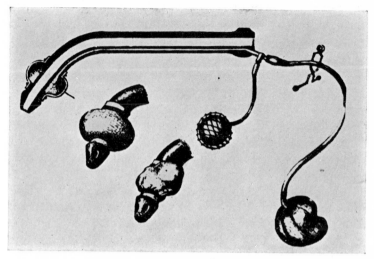

FIGURE 1.—EISENMENGER'S TUBE, 1893

frequency with which a given idea is found to recur in the history of medicine. Usually those who "re-discover" the idea do so in perfectly good faith, unaware that similar work has been done before. Two striking examples of this are to be found in the history of endotracheal anaesthesia. In their paper on the subject, Waters, Rovenstine, and Guedel[13] point out the identical nature of the inflatable cuff of Dorrance,[14] which was described in 1910, and that which Guedel and Waters suggested in 1928[15] without knowledge of Dorrance's work. The inflatable cuff of Eisenmenger is another example of such a "re-discovery." The cuff is shown carrying a bulb on its inflating tube, the tension of the bulb being an index of the degree of inflation of the cuff itself. The same arrangement was suggested by Green[16] in 1906, and within the last three years Hewer[17] has sponsored an identical attachment for use with the cuffs reintroduced by Guedel and Waters.

Work similar to that of Maydl and Eisenmenger was published by Van Stockum of the Hague in 1898.[18] He too was concerned with the prevention of aspiration pneumonia, and he also described a wide-bore tube carrying an inflatable cuff for this purpose. Laryngoscopy was in its infancy at that time, and these tubes were passed through the mouth and inserted into the glottis by touch. Many of these early authors described special curved forceps to hold the tube and facilitate its introduction.

Exactly at the turn of the century Franz Kühn, a surgeon of Cassel, Germany, published the first communication of the series on endotracheal anaesthesia which makes him the outstanding pioneer of that decade. He was aware of the tentative work of Maydl and Eisenmenger, and felt that intubation provided the solution to the problem of anaesthesia in operations upon the upper air passages, by "bringing the air in the trachea into direct contact with the outside air."[19] This would enable the prevention of aspiration, the removal of the anaesthetist from proximity to the field of operation, and the protection of the sterile field from contamination. Kühn suggested a tube made of a coil of flat metal[19] because this material would remain patent under all circumstances, and allowed the tubes to be made with thinner walls. He had meditated the possibility of trauma from the insertion of so hard an object, but decided that the material made little difference and that the secretion of mucus was a sufficient lubricant to offset this.[20] The tubes were from twelve to fifteen centimetres in length, and were inserted with a curved introducer by the sense of touch alone. Between 1901 and 1911 he made certain improvements in the design of his tube, but its essentials remained the same. He was aware of the possibilities of an inflatable cuff, but apparently always preferred a pharyngeal pack of gauze as a protection against aspiration. Having observed that pharyngitis was almost invariably caused by the use of dry gauze, he recommended gauze soaked in oil.[21] He evidently went to a great deal of trouble to use a large pack which completely filled the pharynx and was even pushed down into the cricoid sphincter of the oesophagus.

In 1902 he published a paper on nasal intubation.[22] He felt that nasal intubation was more nearly physiological than oral, and pointed out that a nasal tube "lies better" and leaves the mouth clear of impediments to operation. A nasal tube cannot be bitten by the patient and can, if necessary, be left in place after operation without interfering with the processes of deglutition. From the fact that he did not stress the nasotracheal technique in his later writings we must conclude that increasing experience caused him to decide that the oral route was better suited to his needs and methods.

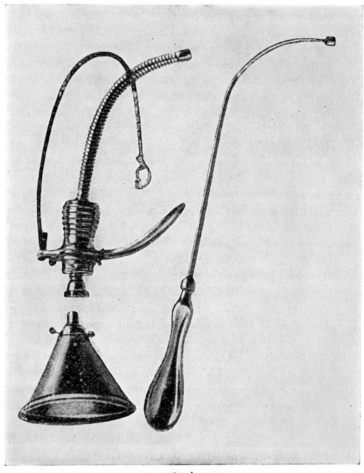

FIGURE 2.—KÜHN'S TUBE, 1902

Showing stylet for its insertion and the elastic band which passed around the neck and held the tube in place.

Kühn appears to have shared the view expressed by Rosenberg[23] in 1895, that the "idiosyncrasy" of some patients to chloroform was due to a reflex arc whose afferent receptor mechanism is situated in the nerve endings of the nasal mucosa. To abolish this Rosenberg recommended the topical application of cocaine to the nose. Kühn felt that cocainization was a helpful adjunct to intubation and frequently used it. He clearly realized (and was, perhaps, the first person to do so) the close relationship between the deficient oxygenation of a patient caused by reflex glottic spasm, and the surgical stimulus in the abdomen which initiates the spasm. He appreciated the fact that a patient's ability to "strain" is diminished when the larynx is mechanically kept open, and as early as 1903 he wrote a paper[24] stressing the improvement in operating conditions in the upper abdomen to be obtained by intubation of the larynx. In two other papers[25, 26] he drew attention to the value of intubation as a resuscitative measure.

Thus far the requirements of the surgeon operating on the head or neck had been the stimulus to the development of endotracheal methods. Curiously enough this statement is true of almost all new developments emanating from Europe. In the United States, on the other hand, the problems of the control of surgical pneumothorax were the chief incentive to research in endotracheal anaesthesia. Perhaps that is why until recently the "low-pressure" inhalation methods were developed in Europe and the "high-pressure" insufflation ones in America. The versatile Kühn, however, was well aware of this other aspect of the question, and devoted both time and thought to it. A series of three articles in the *Deutsche Zeitschrift für Chirurgie* deals with this question.[27] In the first of these Kühn surveys the early literature on intubation for purposes of resuscitation and gives an account of his own work to that date. In the second paper he explains the relation of intubation to the problem of maintaining a sufficient intrapulmonic pressure to prevent the collapse of the lung when the pleural cavity is opened. He describes an apparatus for the administration of chloroform vapor in oxygen under a positive pressure built up by an artificial and controllable obstruction to the exit of vapor from the system. The third paper of this series is especially notable in that it suggests a technique of anaesthesia which was not applied clinically for twenty years, but is now universally accepted: what is now known as the "carbon dioxide absorption technique."*

Kühn had seen machines intended for resuscitation embodying this principle, and felt that such a completely closed system would be the best method for maintaining intrapulmonic pressure. The machine which was then constructed for him closely resembled a modern "circle filter" apparatus. The circle filter contains two canisters filled with solid caustic potash. It was supplied with vapor from a cylinder of oxygen and a chloroform drip-feed apparatus; but the single tube leading to the endotracheal tube from the circle filter, as shown in his illustration, appears to be several feet in length. Since the valves of the circle filter were situated at the machine end of this tube, it follows that there was an enormous dead space in which the patient's carbon dioxide could accumulate. Apparently Kühn was aware of this, for, although he used the machine in experimental animals, he never did so in the human subject. The other reason for its rejection was that he was uncertain as to the possible chemical reactions between the caustic potash and the chloroform.

Thus in the years 1900–1912 Franz Kühn appreciated and applied in practice most of the important points of inhalation endotracheal anaesthesia. His chief weakness was an inadequate appreciation of the importance of minimizing dead space in connecting the endotracheal tube to the source of vapor. Most of his illustrations show lengths of tubing used for this purpose which are incompatible with the efficient elimination of carbon dioxide. This is strange, since he had so clear a grasp of the physiology of respiration and of the necessity of removing this gas. The other criticism which may be directed at his work is that he was not very conscious of minor degrees of trauma re-

---

* This technique, however, had been used by John Snow more than fifty years earlier.

sulting from intubation with a metal tube. He described[28] the use of two tongue forceps "energetically pulled upon" by two assistants; and any worker experienced in Magill's technique of nasal intubation with a rubber tube (see page 83) may well speculate aghast as to the possible consequences of the transnasal passage of an eight-millimetre tube of metal! Kühn dismisses the question of sequelae of intubation by stating that the only complications he had seen were "a slight tenderness and inflammation of the larynx, which disappears in a few hours," and "slight excoriations and haemorrhages which heal quickly." [29] Those workers who have experienced the difficulties of administering anaesthetics for operations in the upper air passages without the aid of endotracheal methods may well sympathize with Kühn's view that the disadvantages of the method were outweighed by its advantages. His work is admirably summarized in his monograph *Die Perorale Intubation*, published in Berlin in 1911. *Littera scripta manent*. Kühn's work is now almost forgotten, but his publications remain the memorial of a man to whose ingenuity and original work anaesthesia owes a great debt.

Thus far all endotracheal anaesthesia had been administered by what is nowadays referred to as the "inhalation" principle (see page 4). The year 1907 saw the introduction of the "insufflation" principle. Barthelemy and Dufour of Nancy,[30] apparently unaware of the work previously done in Scotland, Austria, Germany, and Holland, found this solution to the problem of anaesthesia in operations upon the face. They used the Vernon Harcourt chloroform inhaler as the source of anaesthetic vapor, forcing air through it by means of a hand-bulb. A rubber catheter, of size 18 of the French gauge, was passed into the trachea by touch, and connected to the inhaler by rubber tubing. A dog was first experimented upon, and smooth, uneventful anaesthesia was obtained. Thus encouraged, they satisfactorily anaesthetized an elderly woman for an operation for the excision of the mandible. Although they published an account of only this one case, there is evidence to suggest[31] that they continued to use this method. In spite of the fact that they thus practised, two years earlier, the technique with which Meltzer and Auer (see page 36) are usually credited, they did so empirically. That they did so detracts in no way from the merit of the much more complete investigative work of the latter authors.

While the European workers were seeking to promote smooth anaesthesia in operations upon the upper air passages, those in the United States were chiefly impelled by the requirements of the early workers in thoracic surgery. Parham,[32] in 1898, reported two operations he had performed for the removal of intrathoracic tumors. In his first case the anaesthetic was administered by the time-honored "open mask" technique. The pleural cavity was torn wide open during the operation, and the patient, although he eventually survived, collapsed and almost died at the time. In his second case he used O'Dwyer's modification of Fell's tube[33] for the maintenance of intrapulmonic pressure by the insufflation of chloroform-laden air. The Fell-O'Dwyer apparatus was resorted to when the patient's condition deteriorated upon opening the pleura. A "great improvement" was effected, he tells us. "The assistance rendered by the Fell-O'Dwyer apparatus was evident to all." In 1900 Matas[34] advocated the use of intralaryngeal anaesthesia for the prevention of surgical pneumothorax. He described his modification of the Fell-O'Dwyer apparatus: an endotracheal tube fitted with a plug to occlude the glottic opening so that positive pressure could be exerted through it, and a side-tube to which was attached a funnel of the type used by Trendelenburg for the administration of the anaesthetic. Two papers by Green in 1906[16] and 1907[35] described his experimental methods of anaesthesia for intrathoracic operations in animals. He used a wide-bore tube fitted with an inflatable cuff, and the inflating tube carried a small balloon whose distension served as an index of the inflation pressure of the cuff itself.

In 1909 Meltzer and Auer,[36] two physiologists working at the Rockefeller Institute in New York, published their finding that if air was blown into the trachea of an animal whose respiratory movements had been paralyzed by the administration of curare, full oxygenation of the blood could be maintained. They stipulated that the end of the tube must lie close to the bifurcation of the trachea, that the tube must be narrow enough to permit of the return of the air around it, and that the air must be blown in at a certain positive pressure. They submitted that this method could remove all those difficulties of anaesthesia of which obstruction to respiration was the cause; that herein lay the solution to the problem of regulating the collapse of the lungs in operations involving an open pneumothorax; and that it represented a highly efficient method of artificial respiration. This technique, thanks to the careful and painstaking investigation of its authors, and to its cautious application to clinical anaesthesia by Elsberg,[37] Peck,[38] and many others, achieved rapid success and fame. It has come to be known as "insufflation" endotracheal anaesthesia. Since the principle is dealt with in extenso in Chapter III, its technical aspects will not be dwelt upon here. It increased in popularity so rapidly that by 1913 it was in use in almost all Western European countries as well as in all parts of the United States, and it held the field until 1926.

A few isolated workers continued to use the inhalation principle during this time. Kühn was not to be won away from his advocacy of it. At a discussion held in Berlin in 1910[39] he maintained that the success of his method depended upon the adequate ventilation of the dead space by the patient's own respiratory movements. Meltzer replied that insufflation had the merit that it could ventilate the dead space even in the absence of respiratory movements. Kühn would not believe Meltzer's contention that the return flow of gases in insufflation was of sufficient force to preclude the aspiration of foreign matter into the trachea; Meltzer, on the other hand, did not believe that Kühn's packing of the pharynx could efficiently achieve this end. Kühn therefore, and men influenced by him, such as Kölle,[40] Lötsch,[41] Dirk,[42] Floren,[43] and Köhler[44] continued to use inhalation methods through a wide-bore tube. In 1914 Hill[45] and Mart[46] in England both reported their use of inhalation methods. The former used the term "orotracheal" to describe his route of intubation and stressed the fact that the use of positive pressure was undesirable in other than intrathoracic cases. Mart reported a small series of cases in which he obtained satisfactory endotracheal anaesthesia for oto-rhinological cases by the passage of a wide-bore endotracheal tube. This was provided with a lateral orifice at its proximal end, this end of the tube being open, with the smaller exit tube of a Junker's apparatus leading into it to provide chloroform vapor for the maintenance of anaesthesia. Thus the endotracheal tube served as an airway, and at intervals the lateral hole was occluded by a finger, and chloroform vapor was pumped into the end of the tube by means of the Junker apparatus. This "injection" technique of maintenance of anaesthesia had been suggested and used by Kühn in 1912.[47] Indeed, in this paper he recommended two procedures which have been recently revived. One of these was insufflation by means of a small catheter passed to the bifurcation through his wide-bore tube (see pages 43–45); and he pointed out that this technique could obviate the danger of emphysema if the cords closed in spasm around a single insufflation tube (see page 115). The other was the use of the small insufflation tube for the removal of secretions from the bronchial tree by suction (see pages 151 and 171). In France Guisez[48, 49] took up endotracheal inhalation anaesthesia with chloroform as the solution to the usual technical difficulties encountered in the practice of reconstructive plastic surgery of the face during the first Great War. In the United States Janeway[50] applied Green's experimental methods of anaesthesia to man. In 1913 he described the use of a wide-bore inhalation tube carrying an inflatable cuff for endotracheal anaesthesia with nitrous oxide and oxygen.

With these exceptions, however, until the work of Flagg in the United States, and that of Magill and Rowbotham in England, the insufflation principle was universally used. Kelly,[51] a surgeon of Liverpool, introduced the method into England, where it was developed by Shipway and Boyle, and later by Magill, Rowbotham, and Hewer. Cotton and Boothby[52] and Woolsey[53] advocated the use of mixtures of nitrous oxide and oxygen by endotracheal insufflation in 1911 and 1912 respectively, but this matter did not attract much attention until a decade later. Unger and Bettmann[54] in Germany, and Alessandri[55] and Egidi[56] in Italy all published accounts of their early experiences with insufflation. Endotracheal anaesthesia in any form has never made any headway in the Continental nations since the time of Kühn, probably because of the lack of professional anaesthetists.

During the years 1913–1919 the greatest obstacle to the widespread adoption of endotracheal anaesthesia was progressively overcome. This was the technical difficulty of inserting the tube into the trachea. The art of laryngoscopy was as yet new, intubation having usually been performed by tactile methods with or without the aid of curved introducers or intubating forceps. These were uncertain, and difficulty and failure were frequently encountered. Elsberg[57] however, practised the use of Jackson's direct vision laryngoscope and drew attention to the increase in accuracy and certainty of intubation by this method. In 1913 Chevalier Jackson[58] wrote an article evidently intended for anaesthetists interested in this technique. In it he expressed the view that the larynx should always be examined before intubation in order that any pre-existing disease might be recognized, and that the proper size of tube in relation to the diameter of the trachea might be ascertained. Janeway,[59] in the same year, designed and described a laryngoscope with a curved blade and a dry battery in its handle; but apparently his instrument never achieved the popularity of the Jackson laryngoscope. In this article Janeway stated that some years previously the late T. D. Buchanan had suggested to Jackson the addition of a side-tube to his bronchoscope. This addition made maintenance by insufflation possible during bronchoscopy. During the years 1910–1920 it was gradually realized that the difficulty of intubation varied inversely as the skill and experience of the person performing it.

Evidence progressively accumulated to suggest that the insufflation principle was not all it had originally been hoped to be. Some of its originators' claims on its behalf proved to be exaggerated: the ventilation of the lungs in the absence of respiratory movements was thought to be inadequate, and complications were encountered if an obstruction to the exit of the gases occurred.

The next phase of development arose during and just after the Great War of 1914–1918. The pioneer work of Sir Harold Gillies and his co-workers of the British Army Plastic Unit at Sidcup is now historic in the annals of surgery. No less historic to anaesthetists are the contributions of I. W. Magill and E. S. Rowbotham, the anaesthetists to that unit. They were faced with the problem of providing safe, light, smooth anaesthesia for operations upon the face and upper respiratory passages which frequently lasted several hours; and of being unable to interfere with the patient during this time without contaminating the surgical field. Insufflation endotracheal anaesthesia fulfilled these requirements. A number of interesting points emerged from their work. They found that in these cases it was usually desirable to pass a second tube into the trachea to act as a return airway for the escaping vapor. Not only did this obviate any obstruction to the gas stream, but it also enabled the pharynx to be packed off with gauze. This was a double safeguard against the danger of aspiration, and prevented the blood in the wound from being constantly blown towards the field of operation.[60] The semi-rigid insufflation tubes then in use could be softened by immersion in warm water. These they learned to pass through the nose into the pharynx and thence, by means of a guiding rod[60] or intubating forceps,[61] into the trachea in order that the tube might not impede the surgeon in operations involving the mouth.[62] Since this was a cumbersome proceeding, they presently substituted a wide-bore rubber tube for the second or exit tube. Quite by chance they found that this rubber tube often entered the glottis of its own accord if pushed on through the nose during inspiration; and they realized that the success of this manoeuvre could be recognized by the character of the sounds heard through the tube, and the tactile sensation as it entered the glottis. Obviously, provided the tube was of ample length to reach from the nose through the glottis, if respiration still took place through it when passed into the nose to its full length, it must have lain in the trachea and not in the oesophagus. Further experience convinced them that with increasing practice the majority of patients could thus be intubated "blind"— the term they coined to describe this technique of intubation without recourse to laryngoscopy. This method has, in the intervening years, proved of great value in all cases in which laryngoscopy has been considered inadvisable, and whenever it has been impossible, as in patients with trismus. Magill and Rowbotham had already confirmed for themselves the observation repeatedly made by various workers during the years of the war: that the condition of the patients was more satisfactory after operation if nitrous oxide–oxygen was used for maintenance rather than ether or chloroform.[63] The insufflation of gaseous agents at a positive pressure over long periods of time, however, proved expensive. It then occurred to them that anaesthesia could be more physiologically, as well as more economically, maintained if only one wide-bore rubber tube were inserted into the trachea and the patient were allowed to breathe through it in both directions. This arrangement more closely resembled normal respiration than the forcible insufflation of vapors; it was more economical than the insufflation technique; and the body heat and moisture were better conserved. Thus they reverted to the inhalation principle, to which they adapted the "semiclosed" system of apparatus then recently popularized in the United States by Gwathmey and McKesson, and in England by Boyle.

In the years of "peace" following 1918 the work of Magill and Rowbotham profoundly affected the technique of anaesthesia throughout the British Empire. In all operations upon the head and neck it was found that true asepsis and undisputed possession of his field of work were assured the surgeon by the use of this technique. Inhalation endotracheal anaesthesia gradually supplanted the insufflation methods of Barthelemy and Meltzer by reason of its more physiological character and greater simplicity, and because the danger of producing emphysema was obviated by the fact that in inhalation the gases are delivered to the patient by methods which do not necessitate the use of positive pressure. The trend of papers published on the subject between 1928[62] and 1932[64, 65] makes it evident that there was a gradual transition from true insufflation, through the phase of "inhalation with some degree of insufflation," to pure inhalation. Gradually larger tubes came into use, and smaller rates of flow of the gases—the tendency in this direction receiving fresh impetus from the introduction of the carbon dioxide absorption technique.

In 1924 Waters[66] introduced the "carbon dioxide absorption" technique of anaesthesia, and four years later he and Guedel[15] reminded anaesthetists of the advantages of the inflatable cuff of Eisenmenger and others. The carbon dioxide absorption technique demands a leakproof system for its efficient use, and, when endotracheal methods are desirable, this can best be ensured by the exhibition of an inflatable cuff. The absorption technique, and with it the use of inflatable cuffs and true inhalation endotracheal anaesthesia, achieved rapid popularity in the United States and Canada. In England it made only a few isolated converts, the majority of workers preferring the "semiclosed" method of maintenance of endotracheal anaesthesia through a wide-bore tube. Then, towards the end of 1934, Waters and his associates[67, 68] advocated the merits of cyclopropane as an anaesthetic agent in man. This hydrocarbon gas, being expensive, is most suitably administered by a completely closed technique. It has rapidly found favor both in England and the United States, and has therefore also contributed to the substitution of inhalation for insufflation methods.

The remaining notable advances in endotracheal anaesthesia of recent years have resulted from the new demands made by the rapid advances of thoracic surgery. In the last decade operations for the treatment of bronchiectasis and chronic pulmonary tuberculosis have become commonplace. The patients often exhibit such a quantity of secretion in the tracheo-bronchial tree as may cause death by drowning unless it can be removed during anaesthesia. To meet this difficulty various techniques of drainage by suction either through or outside the endotracheal tube have been devised. A surgeon operating inside the pleural cavity is materially assisted if active respiratory movement can be minimized or abolished while he is actually at work upon the viscera. Such conditions can be provided by the use of the technique known as "controlled respiration" described on pages 111–112. The operations of lobectomy and pneumonectomy are nowadays fairly frequently performed. In the former, infection of the remaining lobe by secretions aspirated from the diseased lobe constitutes a serious risk. Magill[69] has suggested a method of endobronchial suction drainage designed to minimize this risk. Finally, the operation of pneumonectomy is most satisfactorily performed if the main bronchus of the sound side can be intubated with a cuffed tube, so that anaesthesia may be carried on by way of the normal side while the diseased lung is allowed to collapse. This technique of "closed endobronchial anaesthesia" was suggested by Gale and Waters in 1932.[70, 71] It is still *sub judice*, since too few removals of an entire lung have been performed to enable us to form an adequate opinion of its value.

The merits of endotracheal anaesthesia stand established at the present time. Unfortunately any attempt to evaluate its demerits is frustrated by the paucity of recorded fact as to its complications. Certain surgeons and anaesthetists have been prejudiced against the method by a few untoward occurrences which have usually been the fruits of clumsiness or inexperience. The habit of keeping accurate records of clinical experiences is still too rare among anaesthetists. It is to the records to be kept in the future by the rising generation of anaesthetists that we must look for evidence which will enable us to form a more balanced judgment as to the types of patient and operation in which endotracheal anaesthesia should be used.

REFERENCES

1. VESALIUS, A. De Humanis Corporis Fabrica. 1st ed. 1542. p. 658.
2. HOOK, R. Phil. Trans. Roy. Soc. 1667. II. 539.
3. LEROY, J. Jour. de Physiol. 1827. VII. 45.
4. ————Jour. de Physiol. 1828. VIII. 97.
5. MAGENDIE, J. Jour. de Physiol. 1829. IX. 97.

6. SNOW, J.   On Chloroform and Other Anaesthetics. London, 1858. p. 117.
7. TRENDELENBURG, F.   Archiv. f. Klin. Chirurg. 1871. XII. 121.
8. MACEWEN, W.   Brit. Med. Jour. 1880. II. 122 and 163.
9. MAYDL.   Wien. Med. Woch. 1893. XLIII. 57 and 102.
10. O'DWYER, J.   Medical Record, 1887. XXXII. 557.
11. EISENMENGER, V.   Wien. Med. Woch. 1893. XLIII. 199.
12. SHAW, G. B.   The Doctor's Dilemma. Act. I.
13. WATERS, R. M., ROVENSTINE, E. A., and GUEDEL, A. E. Curr. Res. Anaes. & Analg. 1933. XII. 196.
14. DORRANCE, G. M.   Surg. Gyn. & Obs. 1910. XI. 160.
15. GUEDEL, A. E. and WATERS, R. M.   Curr. Res. Anaes. & Analg. 1928. VII. 238.
16. GREEN, N. W.   Surg. Gyn. & Obs. 1906. II. 512.
17. HEWER, C. L.   Recent Advances in Anaesthesia and Analgesia. 3d ed. Philadelphia, 1939. p. 115.
18. VAN STOCKUM, W. J.   Nederl. Tijsch. v. Geneesk. 1898. XXXIV. 179.
19. KÜHN, F.   Zentralbl. f. Chirurg. 1901. XXVIII. 1281.
20. ――――Deut. Med. Woch. 1902. XXVIII. 539.
21. ――――Die Perorale Intubation. Berlin, 1911. p. 146.
22. ――――Münch. Med. Woch. 1902. XLIX. 1456 (Vol. II).
23. ROSENBERG, P.   Berl. Klin. Woch. 1895. XXXII. 14 and 34.
24. KÜHN, F.   Berl. Klin. Woch. 1903. XL. 402.
25. ――――Therap. Monatsh. 1908. XXII. 576.
26. ――――Münch. Med. Woch. 1910. LVII. 1948 (Vol. II).
27. ――――Deut. Zeit. f. Chirurg. 1905: LXXVI. 148; LXXVIII. 467; 1906: LXXXI. 63.
28. ――――Die Perorale Intubation. Berlin, 1911. p. 140.
29. ――――Ibid. p. 155.
30. BARTHELEMY and DUFOUR.   La Presse Medicale, 1907. XV. 475.
31. TUFFIER, Th.   Bull. et Mem. Soc. de Chir. 1914. XL. 557.
32. PARHAM, F. W.   Trans. South. Surg. & Gyn. Assoc. 1898. XI. 223.
33. FELL, G. E.   Buffalo Med. and Surg. Jour. 1887. XXVIII. 145.
34. MATAS, R.   J. A. M. A. 1900. XXXIV. 1371 and 1468.
35. GREEN, N. W. and MAURY, J. W. D.   Ann. Surg. 1907. XLVI. 544.
36. MELTZER, S. J. and AUER, J.   Jour. Exp. Med. 1909. XI. 622.
37. ELSBERG, C. A.   Medical Record, 1910. LXXVII. 493.
38. PECK, C. H.   Ann. Surg. 1912. LVI. 192.
39. KÜHN, F.   Berl. Klin. Woch. 1910. XLVII. 1769 (Vol. II).
40. KÖLLE.   Deut. Zeit. f. Chirurg. 1911. CIX. 98.
41. LÖTSCH, F.   Deut. Med. Woch. 1909. XXXV. 300 (Vol. I).
42. DIRK, A.   Deut. Med. Woch. 1906. XXXII. 1626 (Vol. II).
43. FLOREN.   Therap. Monatsh. 1902. XVI. 507.
44. KÖHLER.   Münch. Med. Woch. 1910. LVII. 2339 (Vol. II).
45. HILL, W.   Proc. Roy. Soc. Med. (Anaes.) 1914. VII. 36.
46. MART, W. D.   Lancet, 1914. II. 1085.
47. KÜHN, F.   Zentralbl. f. Chirurg. 1912. XXXIX. 73 (Vol. I).
48. GUISEZ, V.   Paris Medical. 1916. XXI. 404.
49. ――――La Presse Medicale, 1918. XXVI. 441.
50. JANEWAY, H. H.   Ann. Surg. 1913. LVIII. 927.

51. KELLY, R. E. Brit. Med. Jour. 1912. II. 112 and 617.
52. COTTON, F. J. and BOOTHBY, W. M. Surg. Gyn. & Obs. 1911. XIII. 572.
53. WOOLSEY, W. C. N. Y. State Jour. Med. 1912. XII. 167.
54. UNGER, E. and BETTMANN, M. Archiv. f. Klin. Chirurg. 1913. CI. 118.
55. ALESSANDRI, R. Policlinico, 1912. XIX. 1333.
56. EGIDI, G. Policlinico, 1913. XX. 1769.
57. ELSBERG, C. A. N. Y. State Jour. Med. 1912. XII. 524.
58. JACKSON, C. Surg. Gyn. & Obs. 1913. XVII. 507.
59. JANEWAY, H. H. Laryngoscope, 1913. XXIII. 1082.
60. ROWBOTHAM, S. Brit. Med. Jour. 1920. II. 590.
61. MAGILL, I. W. Brit. Med. Jour. 1920. II. 670.
62. ———Proc. Roy. Soc. Med. (Anaes.) 1928. XXII. 83.
63. MAGILL, I. W. and ROWBOTHAM, S. Proc. Roy. Soc. Med. (Anaes.) 1921. XIV. 17.
64. GRIFFITH, H. R. Curr. Res. Anaes. & Analg. 1929. VIII. 387.
65. TOVELL, R. M. Curr. Res. Anaes. & Analg. 1931. X. 97.
66. WATERS, R. M. Curr. Res. Anaes. & Analg. 1924. III. 20.
67. STILES, J. A., NEFF, W. B., ROVENSTINE, E. A., and WATERS, R. M. Curr. Res. Anaes. & Analg. 1934. XIII. 56.
68. WATERS, R. M. and SCHMIDT, E. R. J. A. M. A. 1934. CIII. 975 (Vol. I).
69. MAGILL, I. W. Brit. Jour. Anaes. 1936. XIII. 92.
70. GALE, J. W. and WATERS, R. M. Curr. Res. Anaes. & Analg. 1932. XI. 283.
71. ———Jour. Thor. Surg. 1932. I. 432.

II. ADVANTAGES AND DISADVANTAGES OF ENDOTRACHEAL ANAESTHESIA

ADVANTAGES

IT IS EVIDENT from the literature that many of the objections expressed in the past have been directed, not at endotracheal anaesthesia itself, but at some particular route or technique of which a given author disapproved. It must therefore be stressed at the outset that this consideration of its advantages and disadvantages applies to any form of endotracheal anaesthesia, provided that it is competently administered.

The arguments in favor of endotracheal anaesthesia fall into three main groups: freedom of airway, the control of intrapulmonic pressure, and artificial ventilation.

FREEDOM OF AIRWAY

Endotracheal anaesthesia procures an absolute freedom of the patient's airway which is mechanically assured. All authorities are agreed that the most frequent cause of difficulty or danger in the administration of an anaesthetic is obstruction of respiration. Intubation removes this cause, and the following advantages result:

With a tube in place in the trachea, spasm of the larynx, should it occur, cannot interfere with the efficacy of respiratory exchange. Laryngeal spasm may be the result of direct irritation of the glottis by too sudden a concentration of a pungent vapor, by a drop of mucus, or by an ill-fitting pharyngeal airway. If its onset is recognized it can usually be abolished by finding the cause and removing it. Once spasm is established, however, intubation is usually the only effective treatment. Reflex glottic spasm is often initiated by surgical stimulus in light anaesthesia, and therefore safety demands either a degree of anaesthesia sufficiently profound to abolish the glottic reflex, or else intubation as a means of maintaining a plane of anaesthesia which is both light and safe. Although any intense surgical stimulus may cause reflex glottic spasm, it occurs most frequently during abdominal operations. Unless the plane of anaesthesia is sufficiently deep to cause paralysis of the glottis, reflex spasm usually results from the stimulus of traction on the peritoneum or of palpation of the structures adjacent to the diaphragm. This spasm, in turn, causes a lack of oxygen which enhances the tension of the unrelaxed muscles, and makes the surgeon's task difficult if not impossible. Until the spasm is relieved and respiratory exchange is re-established it is impossible to deepen the anaesthesia. This vicious circle is familiar to all surgeons as well as to anaesthetists. As long ago as 1903 Kühn[1] pointed out that in abdominal operations intubation promoted smoother anaesthesia, and urged this argument in its favor. Cotton and Boothby[2] were inclined to favor intubation for sub-diaphragmatic operations. Their surmise was confirmed a generation later by Boyle[3] and Hewer.[4] This has in recent years been the common experience of almost all anaesthetists.

If a free airway for the patient is assured, it becomes superfluous for the anaesthetist or his apparatus to remain in close juxtaposition to the patient's head; and he can safely withdraw to a distance without losing anything of his accurate control of the administration, provided that he uses a stethoscope and blood-pressure cuff fitted with sufficient lengths of tubing to permit of close and constant observation of the behaviour of the patient's cardio-vascular system. The movements of the breathing bag will naturally provide him with the necessary information as to the character of the patient's respiration. So long as the anaesthetist's hands and apparatus, neither of which could be kept sterile, perforce encroached on the surgical field at intervals, no true asepsis was possible in any operation upon the head. A tube, once in place, can be treated as part of the surgical field, and remains undisturbed during the operation. In this way endotracheal anaesthesia has made a definite contribution to the recent advances in plastic and cerebral surgery.

In almost all the operations of oto-rhino-laryngology, if anaesthesia by inhalation is employed, a conflict of access to the operative field takes place between the anaesthetist and the surgeon, because the upper air passages are themselves the site of the operation. This very difficulty was the stimulus which excited the work of Kühn, and he solved it by using intubation, as he says,[5] "for the purpose of bringing the air in the trachea into direct contact with the outside air." This "exteriorization of the larynx" enables the surgeon to work unfettered by the necessity either of maintaining a free airway himself or of being interrupted periodically by the anaesthetist's efforts to do so. In certain operations inside the thorax or upon the stomach it is sometimes a help to the surgeon if an oesophageal bougie or stomach tube can be passed. If the patient has been intubated, this can be done without any interruption of the administration of the anaesthetic.[6]

Closely allied to the foregoing advantage is the ability to prevent the aspiration of vomitus, blood, mucus, or pus into the lower respiratory tract. "Aspiration pneumonia" was a fairly frequent sequela of any operation upon the upper air passages in days before intubation was currently used. The aspiration of foreign fluids can always be prevented during operation by the skilful use of endotracheal methods. This fact is of importance not only in operations upon the upper respiratory tract but also in any condition liable to cause the patient to vomit during anaesthesia.

Intubation of the trachea enables the anaesthetist to remove fluids easily, and at any time, from the bronchial tree by suction through or alongside the endotracheal tube. This applies not only to an excess of mucus secreted by the trachea and bronchi, but also to blood or pus. The latter are usually seen only during pulmonary operations, but unless they can be rapidly removed they are a grave menace to the patient. Certain precautions, however, are expedient when applying either negative or positive pressure deep in the respiratory tree (see pages 114–115).

It has long been recognized that certain positions of the patient upon the operating table, although necessary to the operation, greatly impede the mechanics of normal respiration. The chief offenders in this respect are the prone position,[7] the steep "Trendelenburg" position, and any arrangement of the patient which involves the raising of a "bridge" beneath the lower ribs. Not only is respiratory movement hindered, but in these positions it is often difficult if not impossible to prevent upper respiratory obstruction, especially in anatomically "difficult" subjects. Several early workers with endotracheal anaesthesia reported that the incidence of "operative shock" was lower when this technique was in use[8, 9, 10] and suggested that this more favorable condition was due to an absence of exertion during respiration in the intubated patient. Even the very experienced anaesthetist occasionally encounters patients so anatomically abnormal that he is unable to maintain unobstructed respiration with the aid of an artificial airway in the pharynx. In these rare cases intubation will remove the obstruction to respiration where all other measures fail.

Finally endotracheal methods are of great value in those rare cases in which a mechanical obstruction to respiration is either present or anticipated. The least uncommon of these is probably thyroidectomy undertaken for the relief of obstructive symptoms. Naturally intubation must then be accomplished with a tube certain to remain patent under any pressure to which it may be subjected, and of sufficient length to reach beyond the point of constriction of the air passages.

THE CONTROL OF INTRAPULMONIC PRESSURE

If the pleural cavity is opened, the lung which it contains collapses. This collapse can be prevented or remedied by raising the pressure inside the lung. The simplest way to do this is to apply positive pressure to the anaesthetic vapor. The mechanical means of doing so are discussed on pages 112–115 and 153–154. The application of positive pressure can often be achieved by the use of an accurately fitting facepiece. If, however, glottic spasm occurs, or the patient vomits during anaesthesia, it will be impossible to control the intrabronchial pressure. If the glottis is intubated, on the other hand, spasm cannot occur, and vomiting, with suitable precautions, need not disturb the control of the intrapulmonic pressure.

Atelectasis may occur during anaesthesia. If it is diagnosed, the presence of a tube in the trachea renders its immediate treatment possible, by suction drainage of the tracheo-bronchial tree and gentle manual reinflation of the lungs.

The complete collapse of one lung is occasionally desirable during the performance of certain modern operations upon the lung itself. This condition can be secured by the intubation of a main bronchus with a tube carrying a cuff which, when inflated, occludes the bronchus of the diseased side. Respiration is then carried on by the sound lung only (pages 154–156).

The complicated positive and negative pressure cabinets designed for the purpose of preventing pneumothorax during thoracic operations, which enjoyed a considerable vogue at the beginning of this century, have disappeared from use. Increasing experience has thus clearly shown that an appropriate form of endotracheal anaesthesia is both the simplest and the most efficient method of avoiding the difficulties and dangers inherent in the condition of pneumothorax.

ARTIFICIAL VENTILATION

Centuries before the discovery of anaesthesia the resuscitative value of mechanical ventilation was demonstrated (see pages 6–7), and the ability instantly to transmute the maintenance of anaesthesia into the process of resuscitation is a great safeguard to the patient. To such an extent is this true that within the space of a few years the "apnoea" which but recently was the terror of the anaesthetist has under certain circumstances become an accepted technique of anaesthesia.[11] Intubation is no more essential to controlled respiration than to the control of intrapulmonic pressure, for adequate respiratory exchange can usually be effected with a bag and a facepiece. Yet when the maintenance of this exchange is essential to life, and obstruction of the air passages may at any moment interrupt it, intubation offers too valuable a safeguard to be neglected.

Operations in the course of which respiratory failure may occur were formerly embarked upon with trepidation. If intubation is resorted to in such cases, the surgeon can proceed secure in the knowledge that, should respiratory failure occur, the anaesthetist is in a position to substitute effective manual exchange of gases for spontaneous respiration.

Writing at a time when specialist anaesthetists were all but unknown, Kühn said that intubation enabled the surgeon "Herr der Lage zu sein and zu bleiben"[12] (to become and remain master of the field). This is indeed the only possible concise statement of the advantages of intubation: that it makes the anaesthetist master of every mechanical aspect of respiratory exchange, under any circumstances of functional disturbance, and for any period of time.

DISADVANTAGES

The disadvantages of endotracheal anaesthesia are all mechanical. They are inherent either in the act of intubation itself, or in the management of the method when the tube is in place. Intubation is a difficult proceeding which, for its successful accomplishment, calls for the services of a person with special training, skill, and experience. The beginner can acquire the last two qualities only by constant practice. He must at the outset face the fact that learning to intubate is a via dolorosa: that he will often inflict trauma and that he will undergo much embarrassment, vexation, and humiliation in the process of learning. Surgeons should also realize this and should extend to the young anaesthetist the tolerance they exhibit towards the early ineptitude of their own residents. An Australian anaesthetist has drawn a lurid picture of these difficulties: [13] "Being rather an old dog to learn new tricks, my early catheter introductions were along a very blood-bespattered path, slippery with mucus. . . . Ploughing up the pharynx with a laryngoscope in an attempt to dig out an epiglottis from a pool of bloody mucus is one of the least inspiring sights of modern anaesthesia." When Tuffier saw intubation practised in New York he was so impressed with its difficulties that after his homecoming he expressed the view that the method would always be limited in its application because of the mechanical difficulty of passing the tube.[14] In the intervening years his prediction has proved correct in those countries where no medical men have devoted their whole time to anaesthesia. In the United States, however, and throughout the British Empire an ever-increasing interest in anaesthesia has produced a number of anaesthetists capable of skilful intubation. As in all mechanical arts, the acquisition of skill chiefly demands assiduous practice and constant effort to ascertain the causes of difficulty and the methods of overcoming them. Almost all the sequelae of endotracheal anaesthesia are the direct result of a lack of skill in the management of the method, and can be minimized by the acquisition of greater skill and experience.

Intubation, however (except when the blind nasal technique is used), demands anaesthesia sufficiently deep to cause complete relaxation of the mandible and an absence of the pharyngeal and preferably also of the laryngeal reflexes. This state represents a deeper plane of anaesthesia than is necessary for the performance of many of the operations in which endotracheal anaesthesia is desirable. In certain cases, therefore, it is an open question whether the advantages derived from intubation justify the deeper anaesthesia necessary for its establishment.

Intubation involves a greater length of time spent in the induction of anaesthesia. That this is time well spent in view of the improvement subsequently apparent in the operating conditions is not always evident to an impatient surgeon. This disadvantage, again, is largely a matter of skill, since an experienced anaesthetist can perform induction of anaesthesia and intubation in the time required by a novice to achieve the former.

The decision to intubate a patient should be made only after a careful consideration of all these factors. One other point remains. Bitter experience soon teaches the young anaesthetist that there is a certain analogy between skill in playing golf and skill in the administration of an anaesthetic: in both the ability never to get into difficulties is of much greater value than the power of masterly recovery from them. It is obvious from the above recapitulation of its advantages that intubation can preclude many serious difficulties which may arise in the course of administration of an anaesthetic. It has also been pointed out that the technique of intubation is usually not easy. It will be more rather than less difficult in the middle of an operation when undertaken for the urgent relief of an obstruction which has already been allowed to occur. It is therefore probably wise to regard intubation in the light of prophylaxis rather than treatment, and to perform it at the end of induction in cases in which it is felt to be expedient. At any time intubation may become essential during operation because of some unforeseeable complication. When this occurs it often interrupts the smooth course of the operation itself. Intubation during operation is tantamount to a confession of faulty judgment of that particular case. Maturity of judgment and experience enable an anaesthetist to avoid the use of endotracheal anaesthesia in cases in which it is superfluous, and to intubate at the close of induction the patients in whom it will ensure the smoothness of anaesthesia and operation.

Since the introduction of the tube demands an extra expenditure of time, it is obviously superfluous in very short operations unless gross respiratory obstruction is anticipated. As with all other anaesthetics, it is necessary for the anaesthetist to have a clear idea of exactly what the surgeon proposes to do. A frank discussion of the case with him beforehand will often settle whether or not intubation is advisable.

No evidence is yet available that endotracheal anaesthesia increases the incidence of the major respiratory complications in the postoperative period. Unfortunately this is extremely difficult to determine because those cases in which intubation is of the greatest value are precisely the cases in which, for many other reasons, it is known that these complications most frequently occur. The incidence of minor respiratory complications, such as cough or a slight soreness of the pharynx, is probably slightly higher after endotracheal anaesthesia. This, however, is almost entirely a matter of skill in intubation, and varies accordingly.

REFERENCES

1. Kühn, F. Berl. Klin. Woch. 1903. XL. 402.
2. Cotton, F. J. and Boothby, W. M. Surg. Gyn. & Obs. 1911. XIII. 572.
3. Boyle, H. E. G. Brit. Jour. Anaes. 1923. I. 131.
4. Hewer, C. L. Curr. Res. Anaes. & Analg. 1926. V. 303.
5. Kühn, F. Zentralbl. f. Chirurg. 1901. XXVIII. 1281.
6. Quinby, W. C. Med. Comm. Mass. Med. Soc. 1911. XXII. 143.
7. Elsberg, C. A. Ann. Surg. 1911. LIII. 749.
8. Robinson, S. Surg. Gyn. & Obs. 1913. XVI. 296.
9. Peck, C. H. J. A. M. A. 1913. LXI. 839.
10. Coburn, R. C. N. Y. Med. Jour. 1914. XCIX. 1238.
11. Guedel, A. E. Anaesthesiology, 1940. I. 13.
12. Kühn, F. Archiv. f. Rhinol. u. Laryngol. 1911. XXV. 95.
13. Moss, M. K. Curr. Res. Anaes. & Analg. 1930. IX. 168.
14. Tuffier, Th. Bull. et Mem. Soc. de Chir. 1914. XL. 361, 393, and 556.

III. INSUFFLATION
ENDOTRACHEAL ANAESTHESIA

TECHNICAL DETAILS

THE PROGRESSIVE eclipse of insufflation by inhalation methods in the last decade (see pages 21–22) is probably justifiable on physiological grounds. Rare cases sometimes present themselves, however, in which the insufflation technique is of value, and therefore every anaesthetist should be aware of its possibilities and be ready to apply it should it be desirable in a particular case. The following case is a good example of unusual difficulties making insufflation a useful technique:

A young lady of twenty-three was to have all her remaining teeth extracted. Some of these presented abnormalities seen in the radiograph which made a prolonged intervention probable. Her general condition was good, but she had suffered for years from lupus vulgaris. This condition had caused the complete disappearance of her nose, the position which it had occupied being marked only by scarring and by the two small apertures of the nares, both being about 8 millimetres in diameter. The mouth was also contracted by scarring. The anaesthetist was requested to avoid laryngoscopy if possible, since the angles of the mouth had only just healed after many years, and it was feared that they would be broken open by the tension on the tissues. The equipment available was a machine of the "semi-closed continuous-flow" type, without cyclopropane or canisters for the absorption technique.

A nitrous oxide-ether induction was performed, and, when first-plane surgical anaesthesia was reached, a No. 2 Magill tube (of 6½ mm. external diameter) about 27 centimetres long was passed into the trachea by the "blind" technique of Magill, through what remained of the left naris. The expiratory valve of the machine was then tightly closed, and the flow of gases adjusted so that the very thin rubber breathing bag remained full during inspiration. Anaesthesia was maintained with nitrous oxide and 18 per cent oxygen. When the mouth was opened by the dentists, the anaesthetist placed a light gauze pack between the pillars of the fauces, making sure that the return airway through the nasopharynx was unobstructed. This, therefore, was insufflation endotracheal anaesthesia carried out with unorthodox equipment. It provided perfect operating conditions for thirty minutes, and an absence of any sequelae.

As we have seen (page 15), insufflation endotracheal anaesthesia did not originate with Meltzer and Auer, but with Barthelemy and Dufour of Nancy in 1907. To the former workers, however, belongs the credit for the careful investigation of the technique, for their appreciation of its relation to the problem of open pneumothorax, and for painstaking efforts to ascertain its merits and demerits.

Meltzer and Auer[1] defined three conditions which, when fulfilled, enabled respiratory exchange to take place in the absence of respiratory movements. These conditions are as follows: (1) that the lungs are kept in a continuous inspiratory state of distension which facilitates the exchange of gases; (2) that the fresh air reaches the lowest part of the trachea; and (3) that the air escapes by another path than the one by which it enters. They went on to say that "under these conditions the supply of oxygen and removal of carbon dioxide take place apparently in physiological fashion without the aid of any rhythmical antagonistic movement." In their original experiments insufflation was conducted through a tracheotomy opening, but they soon found that a suitable tube passed translaryngeally to the bifurcation of the trachea served their purpose equally well.

The work of the early clinical users of the insufflation method brought out the following points:

That the tube passed should have a diameter from one-half to two-thirds that of the glottic opening.[2] If it was too large, cyanosis tended to occur. If it was too small, it was found difficult to maintain a sufficiently profound level of anaesthesia.

The position of the tube in the trachea was of great importance: the end had to lie within five centimetres of the bifurcation. Otherwise gaseous exchange was deficient, and the patient showed cyanosis.[2] To ensure this depth Meltzer[3] recommended passing the tube until a feeling of resistance indicated its contact with the wall of a small bronchus. It was then withdrawn five or six centimetres. This technique also ensured that the tube was in the trachea and not the oesophagus.

PHYSIOLOGICAL AND MECHANICAL CONSIDERATIONS

It soon became evident that, in spite of Meltzer's original view, the entire suppression of respiratory movement was undesirable. In 1910 he recommended[4] that cyanosis, should it occur, be treated by an interruption of the entering air stream, thus allowing a momentary collapse of the lungs. Almost all the early clinical workers[5, 6, 7] appeared to feel that these periodic interruptions of the entering air stream were important. In 1911 Meltzer[8] suggested that this end could be equally well achieved by constricting the trachea around the tube and thus impeding the return airway. Pauchet,[9] who had evidently studied the work in the United States at first hand, thought that asphyxia could be prevented by producing either further distension or collapse of the lungs. Rosenthal[10] very ingeniously suggested that the difficulty could be overcome by using constant insufflation at a moderate positive pressure of air supplied by a mechanical blower, and supplementing this pressure at intervals by pressing upon a hand air-bulb connected to the tube. This "extra" intermittent pressure would cause an intermittent hyper-distension of the lungs, and therefore artificial pulmonary ventilation. Janeway[11] found, in experimental animals, that hyperpnoea rather than apnoea occurred unless the volume of the lungs was periodically altered by variations of the intrabronchial pressure. Clinically, as Coburn[12] pointed out, it seems evident that some movement of the lungs is necessary to ensure adequate gaseous exchange in the blood.

Such physiological evidence as is available suggests that it is difficult to avoid disturbances in both the oxygen and carbon dioxide content of the blood when using the insufflation technique. In the course of a paper read before the Section of Anaesthetics of the Royal Society of Medicine[13] Pembrey claimed that a total insufflation of thirty litres a minute of air would produce an apnoea during which the blood carbon dioxide tension was lowered. In the discussion of this paper Marshall pointed out that a rise of blood pressure was usually seen during apnoea, and suggested that this might be due to a rise in the carbon dioxide content of the blood. Recent experimental work by Crafoord[14] supports this view. Hirschmann,[15] in 1926, found that there was an increase in the carbon dioxide content of the blood during insufflation. He felt that the apnoea seen during insufflation—to put it in modern terms—depended rather on a preternaturally high threshold of the respiratory centre due to an excess of anaesthetic drug than on a lowered stimulus due to depletion of the carbon dioxide in the blood. He found that the oxygen content of arterial blood was decreased during insufflation, an observation which had already been recorded by Lapeyre[16] in 1917. It appears, then, that the original claims of Meltzer and Auer respecting the efficiency of ventilation by insufflation in a state of apnoea were exaggerated, and that increasing experience caused them to modify their original view. That such an apnoea is due to acapnia is also uncertain. Harris[17] has suggested that it may be due to an interference with the Hering-Breuer reflex resulting from the continuous partial distension of the lungs. It seems obvious that since the changes in intrathoracic pressure resulting from respiratory movement are known to assist the circulation of the blood, any suppression of them will handicap the efficiency of the circulatory system.

Meltzer claimed that in insufflation the return current of air was of such force as completely to preclude the entry of foreign substances into the lower respiratory tract. He and Githens[8] placed charcoal in the stomachs of dogs which were then anaesthetized by the insufflation technique and caused to vomit by means of apomorphine. No traces of the charcoal were found in the trachea. This work was accepted by most of the clinical users of insufflation in the early years,[18] and it is undoubtedly true that a sufficiently forcible current of air returning through the glottic opening will discourage the entry of foreign fluids, and may even serve to blow out a blood clot from the tracheo-bronchial tree.[19] It is debatable, however, whether this safeguard is as reliable as the pharyngeal packing advocated by Kühn or Magill, or the inflatable cuffs of Eisenmenger or Guedel and Waters (see pages 9–10), a possibility which was never appreciated by most of the exponents of the insufflation technique. In 1914 Jeger[20] found insufflation an insufficient guarantee against aspiration and suggested the use of a double insufflation tube fitted with an inflatable cuff. This both safeguarded the return airway and offered absolute protection against aspiration.

DANGERS AND SEQUELAE

It gradually became apparent that certain dangers and inconveniences might result from the insufflation of gases under pressure. First, a sudden increase in intra-alveolar pressure resulting from obstruction to the return flow of the gases might be dangerous. It was found that if pharyngeal obstruction occurred, or the sudden onset of laryngeal spasm blocked the return airway around the tube, the pressure in the lungs naturally rose. This could lead either to alveolar or to surgical emphysema, or both,[21] and it was suggested that the latter was more likely to occur if the tracheal mucosa had been traumatized during intubation.[22] Woolsey,[23] in 1912, mentioned two cases of alveolar rupture and one of emphysema, and Luke[24] reported a case of gross emphysema resulting from the obstruction of the return airway during a cerebellar exploration. It was for this reason that most of the authors who designed machines for insufflation insisted upon the importance of incorporating in them a blow-off valve. Its function was to prevent the pressure from reaching a height which might endanger the lungs should some unexpected resistance to the free exit of the gases arise.

Secondly, structures other than the lungs could be injured by an excess of pressure. It was found that if a high insufflation pressure was used, or if obstruction to the return airway above the glottis occurred,[16] air was forced through the oesophagus and tended to cause a distension of the stomach. This did not endanger the patient—unless a cautery were used upon the stomach in the presence of inflammable vapors—but it did inconvenience a surgeon in the performance of an abdominal operation. Kelly[22] mentioned the use of a stomach tube to prevent this distension. If an insufflation tube is placed in the oesophagus by mistake, however, the stomach may become greatly distended and may even be ruptured by sufficiently high pressures. One death has been caused by this error:[25]

A young adult was to undergo tonsillectomy. "Endotracheal anaesthesia" had, supposedly, been instituted. Just before the operation began the anaesthetist noticed that the patient was slightly cyanotic and that the oxygen cylinder was exhausted. Fine adjustment, but not pressure-reducing, valves were in use on the cylinders. The anaesthetist turned on a fresh cylinder. Unfortunately the fine adjustment valve was open when the main valve was turned on. The compressed gas rushed out with a hiss, and the surgeon, standing by the patient's side, saw the epigastrium rapidly become distended and then suddenly collapse. He announced that he would abandon the tonsillectomy and would perform laparotomy. On opening the abdomen a large hole was found in the cardia: a rupture of the stomach due to the high pressure of the gas. It was repaired as completely as possible, but the patient died of peritonitis early in the post-operative period.

Thirdly, when an endotracheal tube is in place, and the protective closure of the glottis is thereby inhibited, it is inevitable that any pressure applied within the respiratory tract will entail an increase in the intrathoracic pressure. The consequences of this increase are considered in Chapter VI.

AGENTS

Any volatile anaesthetic agent may be administered by endotracheal insufflation. Ether was almost universally used by the early workers in the United States, but almost all the Continental authors used chloroform, and two successful series of cases with this agent were reported in England.[26, 27] American anaesthetists appeared to feel that the danger of overdose with chloroform was too great to warrant its exhibition[6] and that, by reason of its irritancy, it was likely to produce local lesions in the trachea or alveoli.[8] It would seem that experience in the administration of chloroform by other methods reduces the former possibility to a minimum; as for the latter, chloroform is rarely used nowadays except as an adjuvant to mixtures of nitrous oxide and oxygen.

In the early days of insufflation several workers reported the merits of a technique which consisted of an induction with nitrous oxide and sufficient ether to provide the relaxation necessary for intubation.[23, 28] Maintenance could then often be achieved with nitrous oxide and oxygen alone. If this proved impossible, small amounts of ether were added when necessary. This technique was extensively used after the Great War and proved superior to the use of ether or chloroform alone.[29] The insufflation of gases at a positive pressure, however, is an extravagant method of maintenance, especially since, when using agents of marginal potency, the rate of flow must be sufficiently high to preclude the entry of any air during inspiration. Gradually it was realized that more satisfactory anaesthesia and greater economy could be achieved during maintenance if a wider tube were passed and the gases were supplied to it at a low pressure from a tube fitted with a reservoir bag, so that a certain amount of re-breathing could take place. A moderate insufflation pressure was used, and some leakage of the gases occurred between the tube and the walls of the trachea. This lowering of the insufflation pressure and provision for to and fro respiration (or "re-breathing") marked the beginning of the transition from insufflation towards inhalation mentioned on page 22.

APPARATUS

The equipment required for insufflation endotracheal anaesthesia differs slightly from that suited to inhalation methods. The machine should be capable of propelling a stream of air or oxygen through a catheter at a pressure of twenty-five millimetres of mercury, having on the way passed through or over the surface either of ether or of chloroform. The simplest source of gas is a cylinder in which it is stored at a high pressure. To minimize the risk of accidents these cylinders should be fitted with valves which will reduce the delivery pressure of the gases to thirty to sixty pounds per square inch. The exit tube of the machine should be provided with a trap bottle to preclude the possibility of delivering liquid ether or chloroform to the patient. One death has been recorded from this cause.[30] If the anaesthetic gases are to be used, flowmeters should also be fitted to the machine so that the rates of flow can be measured. Either the machine should be provided with a safety valve which can be adjusted to blow off at any desired pressure, or a very light rubber bag should be connected to the tubing running to the catheter. Such a bag should be sufficiently thin to burst before the pressure inside it reaches twenty-five millimetres of mercury.

Anaesthesia may be induced by any agents or techniques which will ensure complete relaxation of the mandible and the opening of the vocal cords widely at each breath. Laryngoscopy is then performed, as described in Chapter V, and a tube of such a thickness as to occupy between one-half and two-thirds of the glottic opening is passed through the open cords and into the trachea. It is gently pushed down until a definite resistance is encountered, and then withdrawn five or six centimetres.[3] If there is any doubt as to the patency of the return airway during maintenance, a second tube of similar size should be passed. This, however, need only lie with its end just below the glottic opening. A rubber tube of appropriate size will perfectly serve this purpose. Rowbotham[31] devised an ingenious method of cutting the end of this tube so that it could be attached to the insufflation tube and be passed with it, and Magill[32] suggested a method of wiring the return tube to the insufflation tube. Eventually a double catheter was put upon the market to simplify the problem of the return airway.

The tubes used for insufflation are usually made either of soft rubber or of semi-rigid composition materials, and may have either a lateral or a terminal opening. The rubber tubes, being soft, require the use of a stylet or a pair of intubating forceps (Figure 15 on page 58) for their insertion, since otherwise the end of the tube cannot be directed anteriorly into the glottic opening. This fact makes them difficult of insertion.[33] Meltzer[3] felt that a tube with a terminal opening was more

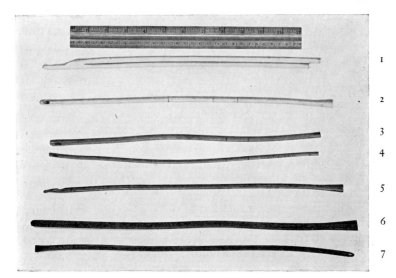

FIGURE 3.—TYPICAL INSUFFLATION TUBES

1. Double Insufflation Tube. 2. White with Lateral Eye. 3 and 4. Semi-Rigid with Terminal and Lateral Eye. 5. Semi-Rigid with Olivary Tip and Lateral Eye. 6 and 7. Rubber with Lateral Eye. F28 and 20.

efficient than one with a lateral opening, and Shipway[34] suggested that tubes with a lateral aperture should be passed with the opening uppermost "so that ether vapor may not be in too close contact with the mucous membrane." Typical insufflation tubes are shown in Figure 3.

Should nasotracheal insufflation anaesthesia be desirable, the tube or tubes are passed through the nose into the pharynx. Laryngoscopy is then performed, and the tips of the tubes are picked up in the pharynx by means of intubating forceps and guided into the glottic opening.[29] Semi-rigid tubes can be softened by immersion in warm water so as to permit of this.

A recent case report by Waters[35] has suggested a modern variant of endotracheal insufflation which can be useful where insufflation is desirable, and which is free of the danger of raising the intrabronchial pressure unduly.

A man of forty was to undergo abdominal exploration for pyloric ulcer. A double indwelling gastric tube was already in place, passing through the nose. Cyclopropane anaesthesia was induced. Orotracheal intubation proved difficult as a large cuffed tube jammed in the small laryngoscope available. A No. 8 Magill tube without a cuff was therefore inserted. As the presence of the gastric tube in the naris precluded an accurate apposition of the facepiece, the smallest size of child's mask was fitted over the lips and the end of the tube, and anaesthesia was maintained for a while by "to and fro" carbon dioxide absorption tech-nique. After thirty minutes the patient's chart showed the signs of deficient ventilation and accumulation of carbon dioxide. The small facepiece did not fit sufficiently accurately to permit of manual augmentation of respiratory exchange. Therefore a No. 18 French gauge rubber catheter was passed through the Magill tube to the bifurcation of the trachea and connected to the exit tube of the gas machine. Ether and oxygen were then insufflated through this small catheter at a small positive pres-sure. This produced satisfactory anaesthesia, and a return of the blood pressure and respiratory rate to normal levels. The respiratory movements were not abolished.

This form of insufflation is probably the safest and most satisfactory technique. By passing the insufflation tube through a Magill tube already in the trachea a free exit for the return-ing gases is assured without the inconvenience of a double in-tubation of the glottis. The danger of emphysema can thus be avoided. Since a Magill tube can usually be passed into the trachea through the nose in light anaesthesia without laryngo-scopy, this technique makes it possible to combine the advan-tages of "blind" intubation with those of insufflation.

"REVERSE INSUFFLATION"

Waters (*loc. cit*) has recently pointed out that alveolar ventilation can be equally well achieved if a catheter is passed to the bifurcation through a Magill tube already in place in the trachea, and connected to a source of suction. Anaesthetic vapor is then supplied around the external orifice of the Magill tube. The result is that this vapor is sucked into the Magill tube, is delivered at the bifurcation, and is sucked out again through the catheter. Under these circumstances, even in the absence of respiratory movements, ventilation can be maintained for short periods. Meltzer was under the impression that suction could not replace positive pressure as the source of ventilation.[4] Waters has, however, encountered rare thoracic cases in which this "reverse insufflation" has proved to be a life-saving measure. As the anaesthetic gases are rapidly removed from the system by the suction, a rapid rate of flow of the gases is necessary as they are supplied to the endotracheal tube.

REFERENCES

1. MELTZER, S. J. and AUER, J. Jour. Exp. Med. 1909. XI. 622.
2. ELSBERG, C. A. Ann. Surg. 1911. LIII. 161.
3. MELTZER, S. J. J. A. M. A. 1914. LXII. 1547.
4. ———Medical Record, 1910. LXXVII. 477.
5. ELSBERG, C. A. Archiv. f. Klin. Chirurg. 1911. XCVI. 57.
6. COTTON, F. J. and BOOTHBY, W. M. Ann. Surg. 1913. LVII. 43.
7. RICKETTS, B. M. Medical Record, 1914. LXXXVI. 505.
8. MELTZER, S. J. J. A. M. A. 1911. LVII. 521.
9. PAUCHET, V. La Clinique, 1911. VI. 120.
10. ROSENTHAL, G. Bull. Gen. de Ther. 1914. CLXVII. 511.
11. JANEWAY, H. H. Ann. Surg. 1914. LIX. 628.
12. COBURN, R. C. N. Y. Med. Jour. 1914. XCIX. 1238.
13. PEMBREY, M. S. Proc. Roy. Soc. Med. (Anaes.) 1914. VII. 34.
14. CRAFOORD, C. On the Technique of Pneumonectomy in Man. Stockholm, 1938. pp. 58-62.
15. HIRSCHMANN, C. Beitrag. z. Klin. Chirurg. 1926. CXXXVII. 248.
16. LAPEYRE, C. Jour. de Phys. et de Path. Gen. 1917. XVII. 219.
17. HARRIS, T. A. B. Brit. Med. Jour. 1935. I. 129.
18. SHIPWAY, F. E. Proc. Roy. Soc. Med. (Anaes.) 1914. VII. 31.
19. MAGILL, I. W. Proc. Roy. Soc. Med. (Anaes.) 1930. XXIII. 778.
20. JEGER, E. Deut. Med. Woch. 1914. XL. 227 (Vol. I).
21. GEORG, C. Am. Jour. Surg. (Anaes. Supp.) 1917. XXXI. 77.
22. KELLY, R. E. Brit. Med. Jour. 1912. II. 617.
23. WOOLSEY, W. C. N. Y. State Med. Jour. 1912. XII. 167.
24. LUKE, H. C. Surg. Gyn. & Obs. 1913. XVI. 204.
25. Referred to by G. EDWARDS. Brit. Jour. Anaes. 1938. XV. 93.
26. MART, W. D. Lancet, 1914. II. 1085.
27. MOTT, C. H. Proc. Roy. Soc. Med. (Anaes.) 1920. XIII. 25.
28. COTTON, F. J. and BOOTHBY, W. M. Surg. Gyn. & Obs. 1911. XIII. 572.
29. MAGILL, I. W. and ROWBOTHAM, S. Proc. Roy. Soc. Med. (Anaes.) 1921. XIV. 17.
30. FISCHER, H. Surg. Gyn. & Obs. 1911. XII. 476.
31. ROWBOTHAM, S. Brit. Med. Jour. 1923. I. 1090.
32. MAGILL, I. W. Lancet, 1924. I. 1320.
33. TUFFIER, Th. Bull. et Mem. Soc. de Chir. 1914. XL. 556.
34. SHIPWAY, F. E. Brit. Med. Jour. 1913. II. 1621.
35. WATERS, R. M. Minutes Anaes. Staff Meetings, Wisconsin General Hospital, December 18, 1940 (unpublished).

IV. EQUIPMENT AND APPARATUS FOR INTUBATION

INSUFFLATION endotracheal anaesthesia having been discussed in the previous chapter, we shall now confine our attention to the inhalation principle. Most of the techniques by which the trachea may be intubated are common both to insufflation and inhalation; certain of them are only practicable with a particular variety of tube.

VARIETIES OF TUBES FOR ENDOTRACHEAL INHALATION

Three materials are commonly used for the manufacture of endotracheal tubes: metal, rubber compositions or woven silk of various types, and rubber.

Metal tubes have the advantage that, being rigid, they cannot be obstructed by kinking; and that, because of the strength of the metal, they can be made with very thin walls, thus minimizing the restriction in size of the glottic opening by their presence. They are very durable and can be sterilized by boiling. A metal tube is thought by most authorities to be potentially traumatic to the delicate mucosa of the respiratory tract, and for this reason the metal tubes used by Kühn fell into disuse until their revival by Flagg[1, 2] in 1929. For purposes of anaesthesia, unlike those of bronchoscopy, the tube cannot well be rigid throughout, and therefore all three varieties of metal tube in current use have a central section of flexible metal hose. To minimize trauma, and to make the metal coils airtight their protagonists recommend that they be covered with thin "Penrose" rubber tubing. Flagg's original tubes were constructed after discussion with Chevalier Jackson because these authorities were convinced that a rigid metal tube was not traumatic, and because it offered the advantages referred to. Flagg's tube is really a flexible modification of the Jackson type bronchoscope. Woodbridge[3] modified the original Flagg tube in 1934 by shortening the solid metal tip so that almost the entire tube consisted of flexible coiled wire. In 1932 Coryllos and McKesson[4, 5] designed a metal tube which was intended for use during thoracic operations. It is similar to the other

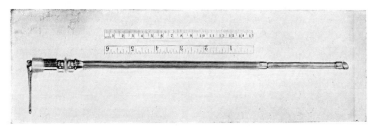

FIGURE 4.—SEVEN-MILLIMETRE FLAGG'S TUBE WITH STYLET IN PLACE

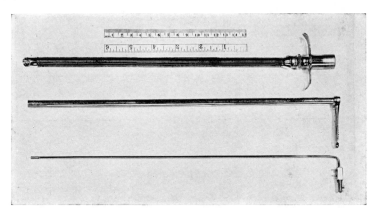

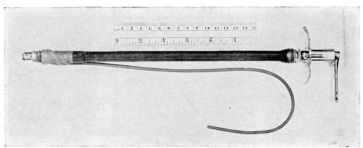

FIGURE 5.—WOODBRIDGE TUBE
Above: Dismantled. *Below:* Assembled with inflatable cuff.

metal tubes, but is provided with distal illumination like a
bronchoscope. Any tube can, however, be illuminated by the
use inside it of a rigid stylet carrying a small bulb of the type
used in distally illuminated bronchoscopes. These three types
of metal tube are shown in Figures 4-6.

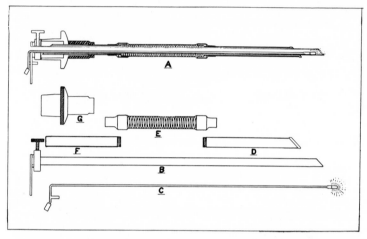

FIGURE 6.—THE CORYLLOS-MCKESSON TUBE

A. The entire instrument. B. The stylet. C. The lamp-carrier. D and
F. The two rigid metal segments of the tube. E. The flexible middle
segment. G. The mouth-prop.

A great variety of tubes made of semi-rigid materials has
been used. Hargrave[6] advocates the use of silver wire covered
with flexible silk elastic, and his wide-bore tubes were originally made with the usual bevelled tip. More recently[7] he has
modified this by lengthening the bevel and attaching an olivary
tip, feeling that this facilitates its passage between the cords.
One London firm manufactures "Chiron" tubes of a semi-rigid
greyish material. Another firm lists three varieties of open-
ended, semi-rigid, wide-bore tubes. Some of these are made of
a white material and are named after F. P. de Caux. The "Anode"
tube is a very soft rubber tube reinforced by a wire spiral
inside the rubber to prevent it from kinking. It is, however, so
flexible that it requires a stylet or a pair of intubating forceps

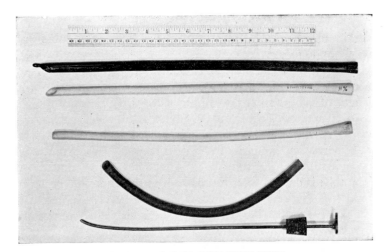

FIGURE 7.—TYPICAL INHALATION TUBES

From the top down: Hargrave's with olivary end. De Caux's. White with open end. Anode with stylet.

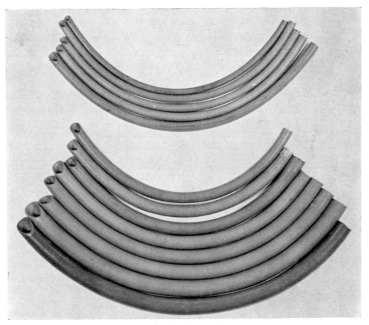

FIGURE 8.—A SET OF MAGILL TUBES

Above: Sizes 00-2 not yet cut down. *Below:* Sizes 3-10 in actual use.

for its insertion. The chief varieties of inhalation tubes are shown in Figure 7.

Finally, there are the curved rubber tubes with which the name of I. W. Magill is associated. These merely consist of a length of rubber tubing with a bevelled tip. Originally Magill used commercial rubber tubing,[8] but the tubes have more recently been made of a special mineralized rubber designed to remain resilient in spite of a very thin wall. This is the only type of tube equally suitable for nasal and for oral intubation. The tube is curved so as to conform to the curve of the nasal fossa (see Figure 28 on page 87), and the bevel is so cut that the point is to the right when the tube is viewed from its concave aspect. Figure 8 illustrates a set of Magill tubes.

The metal tubes are made in sizes varying from 5 to 11 millimetres outside diameter; the others in a wider range from $4\frac{1}{2}$ to $12\frac{1}{2}$ millimetres. Much confusion has arisen because it has been customary to refer to the sizes of bronchoscopes and metal tubes in millimetres, and those of semi-rigid tubes in terms of the "French" catheter gauge, whereas the Magill rubber tubes have been arbitrarily numbered from 00 up to 10. In Table I these sizes have been correlated as nearly as possible by the measure-

TABLE I

A COMPARISON OF THE VARIOUS SCALES OF MEASUREMENT BY WHICH THE SIZES OF ENDOTRACHEAL TUBES ARE STATED

Magill Tube Sizes	"French" Catheter Gauge	External Diameter Millimetres
00	13	$4\frac{1}{3}$
0A	16	$5\frac{1}{3}$
0	17	$5\frac{2}{3}$
1	18	6
2	20	$6\frac{2}{3}$
3	23	$7\frac{2}{3}$
4	25	$8\frac{1}{3}$
5	27	9
6	29	$9\frac{2}{3}$
7	30	10
8	32	$10\frac{2}{3}$
9	34	$11\frac{1}{3}$
10	37	$12\frac{1}{3}$

ment of a large number of tubes. Absolute accuracy is impossible because many of the tubes show individual variations. Any inhalation tube may be fitted with an inflatable cuff as described by Guedel and Waters.[9]

LARYNGOSCOPES

Every anaesthetist should be adept in laryngoscopy and should possess an efficient laryngoscope, irrespective of the frequency with which he practises endotracheal anaesthesia; for in rare cases the ability to examine and intubate the glottis is a life-saving measure.

Chevalier Jackson's laryngoscope[10] is the standard instrument among laryngologists, and has been extensively used by anaesthetists. Unfortunately for the latter, the illumination depends upon a large dry battery from which cords run to the instrument. This makes it cumbersome to carry and use. Moreover, its bulbs are small and fragile, and can on occasion become dangerously hot. One fatal explosion of anaesthetic vapor has resulted from this cause.

The laryngoscopes in common use among anaesthetists fall into two main categories: the "U-type" and the "L-type," so called because of the shape of the instrument. In the former the blade is parallel to the handle; in the latter it is at a right angle to the handle. The U-type have the advantage that they can be grasped either horizontally or vertically, whereas the L-type can be held only in the latter position. They all consist of a blade or speculum, flattened into a smooth beak at the distal end and rounded into a partial tube proximally, and they are provided with an electric bulb which illuminates the region of the beak. The speculum is open on the right side, forming a channel to permit of the passage of the tube. The electric wiring should be so contrived that neither it nor the bulb encroaches upon the lumen of the instrument, thereby obstructing the view or the passage of the tube. In the surgical instruments the speculum is a closed tube provided with a slide that can be removed when it is desired to pass another instrument through the laryngoscope. A removable slide which will occlude the channel is a

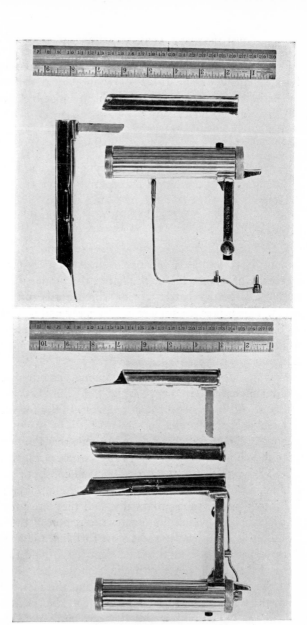

FIGURE 9.—MAGILL'S LARYNGOSCOPE

Above: Dismantled for sterilization. *Below:* Assembled,
showing an interchangeable blade of smaller size.

useful addition to the anaesthetist's laryngoscope: it will prevent the tongue, a single tooth, or a loose premaxilla from bulging into the lumen of the instrument and obstructing the view. Two instruments so provided are illustrated in Figures 9 and 13. The handle of the instrument contains a dry cell which provides the electricity to light the bulb, and there is usually a switch which enables the light to be turned off or on. It is unwise to leave the battery in the instrument when it is not in use, for short-circuits are prone to occur, and switches are easily turned on by accident. Spare bulbs and batteries should always be available, and the instrument to be used should always be tested immediately before beginning the induction of anaesthesia. Most of

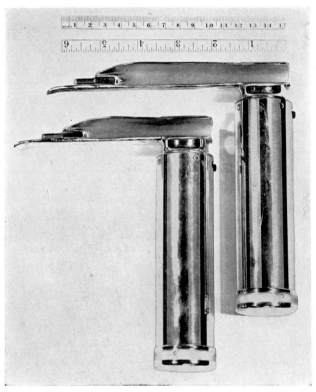

FIGURE 10.—FLAGG'S LARYNGOSCOPE, LARGE AND SMALL

the laryngoscopes illustrated are provided with interchangeable blades of different sizes. Only in certain models, however, can the lighting equipment be removed from the blade and the latter detached from the battery so that it can be boiled. Since laryngoscopes are frequently used in cases showing highly in-

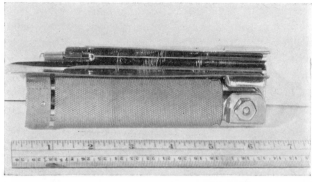

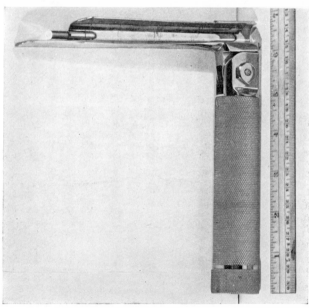

FIGURE 11.—FOLDING LARYNGOSCOPE
Above: Folded. *Below:* Open and alight.

fective organisms, this seems a desirable attribute. Where the instrument cannot be taken apart, the blade is washed after use with soap and water and then immersed in an antiseptic solution for some hours. This solution must be removed from the instrument before the latter is used. Since in large numbers of

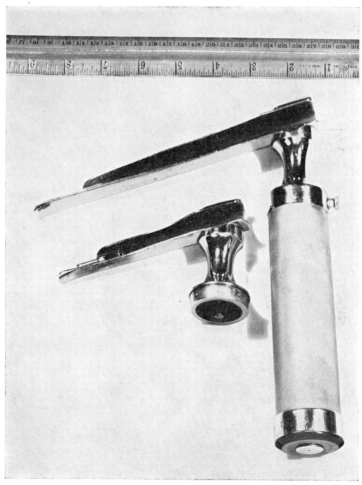

FIGURE 12.—GUEDEL'S LARYNGOSCOPE, SHOWING INTERCHANGEABLE BLADE OF SMALLER SIZE

cases no cross-infection attributable to this method of sterilization has occurred, it is to be inferred that it is clinically effective. But the careless use of liquid antiseptics is apt to corrode the metal parts and promote unexpected failures in the electrical lighting system.

Flagg's laryngoscope[11] (Figure 10) in the United States, and Magill's[12] (Figure 9) in Britain have been the most widely used, and have given rise to a number of modifications. Two of these are illustrated in Figures 11 and 12. The most recent is a folding laryngoscope in which the blade can be folded back so that it lies parallel to the handle (Figure 11). The switch mechanism is so arranged that it makes contact as the blade reaches the right-angle position. This makes the instrument easy to carry and eliminates the danger of wasting the battery when it is not

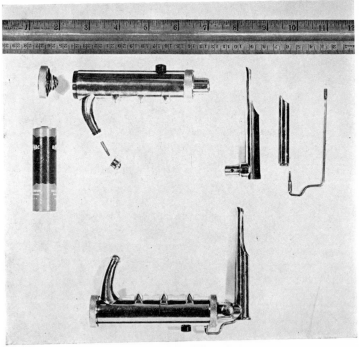

FIGURE 13.—SHADWELL LARYNGOSCOPE

Above: Taken apart for sterilization. *Below:* Assembled.

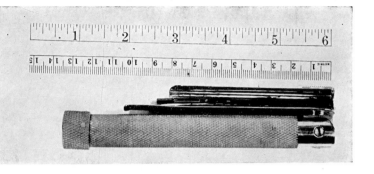

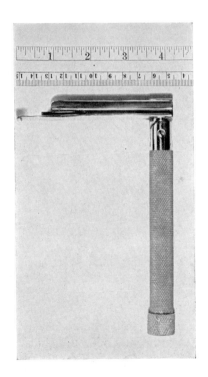

FIGURE 14.—FOLDING LARYNGOSCOPE, SMALL SIZE FOR INFANTS
Above: Folded. *Below:* Open and alight.

57

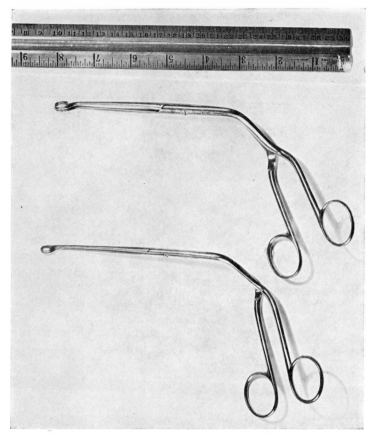

FIGURE 15.—INTUBATING FORCEPS

in use. Neither the blade nor the lighting equipment is removable. In Guedel's (Figure 12) and Goldman's[13] models, both of which are modifications of the L-type, the handle is set at an acute angle to the blade.

Intubation of the very small infant is best performed with a specially designed instrument. Endotracheal anaesthesia is chiefly useful in these subjects in plastic operations on the head or neck. Intubation for the treatment of asphyxia neonatorum is sometimes a life-saving measure which an anaesthetist should be prepared to undertake whenever necessary. Two special infants' laryngoscopes have been designed for these purposes: the "Shadwell" laryngoscope[14] (Figure 13) and a small instrument made at the University of Wisconsin which has not yet been described in print (Figure 14). The former is merely an anaesthetist's modification of the smallest size of Jackson's laryngoscope. The latter is a miniature of the folding laryngoscope previously described.

INTUBATING FORCEPS

Intubating forceps should always be available, although they should rarely be used. They are sometimes necessary to insert flaccid tubes and often useful to persuade a soft gastric tube to pass through the cricoid sphincter into the oesophagus, or to insert pharyngeal packing through a laryngoscope. There are several types of intubating forceps, of which Magill's latest pattern (Figure 15) is probably the most generally useful. It is made in two sizes, the smaller of them being exclusively designed for use with the Shadwell laryngoscope. In infants the mouth is usually too small to permit of digital packing of the pharynx and this is best accomplished by means of the small forceps. Lundy and Tovell[15] have found that the utility of the Magill forceps can be increased by attaching to its blade a laryngoscope bulb which is illuminated by a small dry-cell.

ANGLE-PIECES

Some form of connection or angle-piece is necessary when rubber tubes are in use, to enable the source of anaesthetic vapor to be adapted to the tube. Many forms of these have been devised. Any of the more usual types shown in Figure 16 can be easily and inexpensively made by any competent mechanic. The ideal angle-piece should (1) take so firm a grip of the tube that it cannot slip out during the operation; (2) be of such a width as to cause no narrowing of the lumen of the tube; (3) readily admit of the passage of a suction catheter through the tube; and (4) be of such a shape that it can be easily and firmly secured to the lips, face, or nose by adhesive strapping.

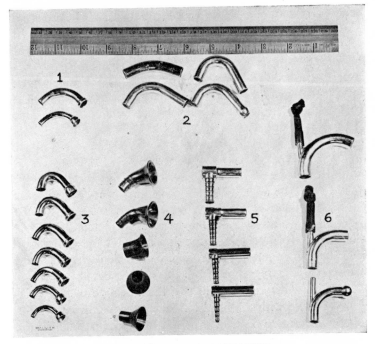

FIGURE 16.—TYPES OF ANGLE-PIECES

1. "Oral" Magill type. 2. Improvised wide-bore type. 3. "Nasal" Magill type. 4. Funnel type. 5. Rowbotham type. 6. Suction type.

The funnel type of angle-piece is intended for use when the tube is passed as a laryngeal airway and is left beneath the anaesthetic mask instead of being connected directly to the gas machine.[16] Its function is to prevent nasal tubes from disappearing into the nose during anaesthesia, and yet not cut the lips or become obstructed against the side of the mask. The angle-piece provided with a side-tube is intended to facilitate the passage of a suction catheter through the endotracheal tube, and was designed primarily for thoracic cases. It is useful in any patient who has excessive bronchial secretion.

CUFFS—PACKING

Certain other pieces of equipment are desirable. If a completely gas-tight endotracheal anaesthetic is desired, an inflatable cuff[9] or laryngeal plug[17] must be used. Cuffed tubes and the syringe and forceps for their inflation are shown below.

When orotracheal intubation is performed the tube must be protected from being bitten by the patient. Various objects placed between the teeth may be used for this purpose: wooden spools, gauze rolls, metal dental props, or mouth gags. A supply of adhesive strapping with which to secure the tube in place after intubation should be available.

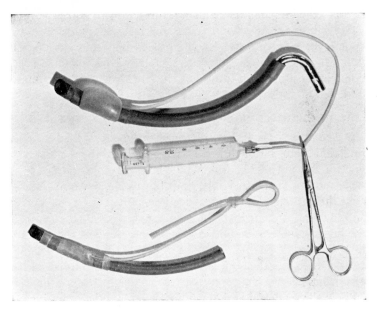

FIGURE 17.—MAGILL TUBES CARRYING INFLATABLE CUFFS: TO SHOW THE METHOD OF INFLATION (see pages 79-83)

If a leakproof system is not essential, pharyngeal packing may be substituted for the cuff or plug. The most usual form of packing consists of a roll or plug of soft gauze impregnated with a lubricant. Dry gauze should never be used because it is abrasive and usually gives rise to pharyngitis in the postoperative period.[18] Magill's method of preparing gauze for this purpose is to fill a clean glass jar with rolls of soft two-inch bandage. A considerable quantity of sterile liquid paraffin is then poured into the jar and is absorbed by the bandages. When intubation has been performed the mouth is opened wide and the gauze is packed into the pharynx gently but firmly around the tube, the roll of bandage being held in a towel by an assistant. The chief objection to this method is the greasiness resulting from the excess of paraffin on the patient's face and the anaesthetist's hands. This can be minimized by keeping the bandages used for packing in a dry jar when once they have become fully impregnated with paraffin. Gauze wet through with saline solution is less abrasive than when it is dry, but its use does not entirely abolish the incidence of pharyngitis. An inflatable pharyngeal cuff around the tube has been suggested by Rowbotham, but it complicates intubation and is less efficient than an endotracheal cuff.[19]

LUBRICATION OF TUBES; LOCAL ANALGESICS

Apparently it was unusual to lubricate the small-bore insufflation tubes, although Pope[20] recommended the use of vaseline for this purpose in 1913. Wide-bore tubes, however, are a trifle more difficult to insert, and lubrication not only facilitates their passage but may reduce irritation of the vocal cords and trachea. Vaseline is used by some workers.[21, 22] It furnishes the greatest lubrication but hastens the perishing of rubber and thus shortens the period of service of rubber tubes and inflatable cuffs. Other workers[23] prefer non-greasy water-soluble lubricant jellies because they feel that vaseline might act as a foreign body in the trachea. Liquid paraffin is used by others, but it also is inimical to rubber. Either vaseline or paraffin might give rise to an "oil pneumonia." Brennan[24] suggested the incorporation of a local analgesic in the lubricant to minimize the coughing which is apt to occur if the tube is moved in the trachea during light anaesthesia, and recommended a lubricant paste having the following composition:

R	Paraffin Dur.	gr. xv
	Cera Alba	gr. xxx
	Paraff. Moll. Alb.	℥ i
	Nupercaine Base	10%

There is also on the market an ointment consisting of a mixture of 1 per cent "Diothane"* in 99 per cent of a bland base which resembles lanoline. Both these preparations are satisfactory as local analgesics, but are deficient in lubricating properties. It will probably prove possible in the future to evolve a combination of these with soft vaseline which will prove efficient both as a lubricant and as an analgesic.

It is often convenient to be able to produce a local analgesia in the nose, pharynx, larynx, or trachea by spraying them with an analgesic solution through a nebulizer. The following substances have been used for this purpose, and have proved satisfactory: Cocaine in solutions varying from 2 to 20 per cent, Nupercaine† in a strength of 2 per cent, Pontocaine‡ in either 1 or 2 per cent solution, Butyn§ in a strength of 1 per cent, and Diothane in a 1 per cent solution. An efficient nebulizer should therefore be available when intubation is to be performed.

If a patient exhibits mucus, pus, blood, or vomitus in the pharynx during induction, these should be removed before intubation. It is therefore a convenience to the anaesthetist if suction is provided in the anaesthetizing room. If this is not available, the pharynx must be cleaned out with small gauze swabs held by an intubating forceps.

THE CARE AND STERILIZATION OF TUBES

It seems appropriate to close a chapter devoted chiefly to apparatus and equipment with a few remarks on this subject, on which little has ever appeared in print, for the point is of some interest, to judge by the discussions that often take place between individual workers.

Tubes of all types should be cleaned out thoroughly as soon as possible after use. A test-tube brush of appropriate size[25] should be used with warm water and soap. There is usually mucus and sometimes blood in the lumen of the tube, which

---

* Piperidinopropanediol di-phenylurethane hydrochloride.
† Alpha butyl oxycinchoninic acid diethyl ethylene diamide hydrochloride.
‡ Para butyl amno benzoyl dimethyl amino ethanol hydrochloride.
§ Para amino benzoyl gamma dinormal butyl amino propanol sulphate.

either heat or antiseptics will coagulate and make difficult to remove. Water should not be allowed ingress into an inflatable cuff, and the inflating tube should be tied or clamped off during the process of washing. Any lubricant remaining on the tube is then removed with a towel soaked in ether. Metal tubes can then be boiled, provided no electrical fittings are boiled with them. The semi-rigid tubes and rubber inflatable cuffs are ruined by boiling and must therefore be sterilized by immersion in a weak antiseptic solution. A 1:1000 solution of mercury biniodide and strengths of alcohol varying from 60 to 90 per cent are commonly employed for this purpose.

The care as well as the sterilization of the rubber Magill tubes is a controversial subject. Having used the identical tubes extensively both in England and in the United States the author ventures to propound the following views. It is not generally realized that for consistent success in nasal intubation by the "blind" technique of Magill (see page 83) the shape of the tube is of considerable importance. It should be curved in the antero-posterior plane, a shape which also facilitates orotracheal intubation. The exact degree of this curve varies with the position of the head preferred by the individual worker: the greater the flexion of the patient's head the more acute should be the angle of the curve. Unless these rubber tubes are kept in a circular receptacle they tend to lose this curve, and Adams[26] has designed special curved glass containers in which the tubes are kept sterile ready for use. The author's personal preference is best served by the curve produced when the tubes are kept in a circular tin box measuring seven and a half inches in diameter. The tin box is lined with a sterile towel and passed through the autoclave. The tubes are then boiled for about ten minutes and placed in the curve of the box with sterile forceps. Dipping them for a moment in 90 per cent alcohol when withdrawn from the sterilizer appears to help maintain their stiffness. An effort is then made to avoid handling the tracheal end of the tube when withdrawing it from the box for use. Many American and some British workers object to this method on the ground that repeated boiling causes the tube eventually to become soft and useless. This fate ultimately over-takes all Magill tubes however they are sterilized. In comparing the condition of tubes used under identical conditions in the same institution, but sterilized by the two different methods, there has been no perceptible difference in the rate at which they either became soft or perished. It is true that rubber de-teriorates more rapidly in the United States than in England, probably because of the much higher indoor temperature and lower humidity. Whether a Magill tube is boiled or sterilized by immersion in antiseptics, its "life," if used three times a week, is probably not longer than three or four months.

Magill[25] insists that angle-pieces be removed from his tubes before they are cleaned, since if left in place they eventually distend the proximal end of the tube. His own practice is to boil a tube for two minutes before using it, and place it in a 1:1000 solution of biniodide of mercury. The excess of this solu-tion is then shaken off before the tube is passed. If different types of angle-piece are to be used, their removal after each case is essential. The alternative is to leave the angle-piece in situ during the entire "life" of the tube. This results in a very firm attachment of the tube to the angle-piece.

Magill tubes are sold in lengths of over thirty centimetres, the intention being that they be cut down to suit the require-ments of the individual patient. The great initial length per-mits of their use for endobronchial intubation. A new tube, therefore, should not be used until its length has been meas-ured (see pages 104–105).

REFERENCES

1. FLAGG, P. J. Laryngoscope, 1929. XXXIX. 594.
2. ————Curr. Res. Anaes. & Analg. 1929. VIII. 327.
3. WOODBRIDGE, P. D. Curr. Res. Anaes. & Analg. 1934. XIII, Supplement, p. 68.
4. CORYLLOS, P. N. Curr. Res. Anaes. & Analg. 1932. XI. 138.
5. ————Jour. Thor. Surg. 1933. II. 384.
6. HARGRAVE, R. Curr. Res. Anaes. & Analg. 1929. VIII. 103.
7. ————C. M. A. J. 1932. XXVI. 218.
8. MAGILL, I. W. Brit. Med. Jour. 1930. II. 817.

9. GUEDEL, A. E. and WATERS, R. M. Curr. Res. Anaes. & Analg. 1928. VII. 238.
10. JACKSON, C. Bronchoscopy, Oesophagoscopy & Gastroscopy. 3d ed. Philadelphia, 1934. p. 21.
11. FLAGG, P. J. Arch. Otolaryngol. 1928. VIII. 716.
12. MAGILL, I. W. Lancet, 1926. I. 500.
13. GOLDMAN, V. A. Brit. Med. Jour. 1936. II. 394.
14. GILLESPIE, N. A. Brit. Jour. Anaes. 1939. XVII. 2.
15. LUNDY, J. S. and TOVELL, R. M. Proc. Staff Meetings Mayo Clinic, 1935. X. 257.
16. GILLESPIE, N. A. Lancet, 1934. II. 548.
17. GUEDEL, A. E. Personal Communication.
18. NOSWORTHY, M. D. Theory and Practice of Anaesthesia. 1st ed. London, 1935. p. 135.
19. HEWER, C. L. Recent Advances in Anaesthesia & Analgesia. 3d ed. Philadelphia, 1939. p. 116.
20. POPE, S. T. Calif. State Jour. Med. 1913. XI. 255.
21. MAGILL, I. W. Newcastle Med. Jour. 1934. XIV. 67.
22. TUOHY, E. B. Proc. Staff Meetings Mayo Clinic, 1936. XI. 91.
23. McCARTHY, K. C. Anaesthesiology, 1940. I. 216.
24. BRENNAN, H. J. Lancet, 1938. I. 315.
25. MAGILL, I. W. Am. Jour. Surg. 1936. XXXIV. 450.
26. ADAMS, R. C. Proc. Staff Meetings Mayo Clinic, 1937. XII. 730.

V. INTUBATION

INTUBATION of the glottis is a difficult proceeding, requiring skill born of long experience for its successful performance. Almost all authors in the past have emphasized the fact that deep anaesthesia facilitates intubation, but few have mentioned the desiderata produced by deep anaesthesia. Most techniques of intubation are facilitated by deep anaesthesia; a few are not. The ease or difficulty of intubation depends upon the presence or absence of muscular flaccidity, pharyngeal reflexes and laryngeal reflexes, and upon the rate and volume of respiration. These in turn largely depend upon the smoothness and competence of the induction of anaesthesia to the optimum level. Skilful induction is therefore more important than the act of intubation itself, which the induction can make or mar.

OROTRACHEAL INTUBATION

BY DIRECT LARYNGOSCOPY

Inspection of the radiographs shown in Figures 18 and 19 will reveal the mechanical problems involved. In the normal position of the structures (Figure 18) the line from the upper incisor teeth through the pharynx to the glottis is almost a right angle. This must be converted into a straight line by the laryngoscope to enable the glottis to be seen. To achieve this straight line the base of the tongue and the epiglottis must be lifted anteriorly. Because of variations in structure between individuals, this is comparatively easy to do in most, exceedingly difficult in some, and impossible in certain abnormal subjects. In large plethoric men who have wide and short necks, and in patients with long, high palatal arches, protruding incisor teeth, or short receding mandibles, exposure of the glottis by direct laryngoscopy is difficult. It is usually easy in edentulous patients. Figures 18 and 19 are lateral radiographs of the head and neck taken of patients who had been intubated orally. In

Figure 18 a Magill tube is in place in a patient with normal teeth, whereas in Figure 19 a Woodbridge metal tube is in the trachea of an edentulous patient, and a stomach tube can be seen passing through the nose into the oesophagus. A compari-

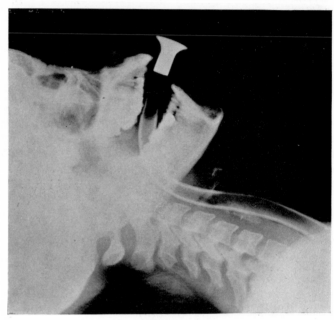

FIGURE 18.—LATERAL RADIOGRAPH OF THE HEAD AND NECK, SHOWING ORAL
INTUBATION IN NORMAL PATIENT WITH MAGILL TUBE

son of these will reveal the greater difficulties of exposure in the first case as compared with the second.

Before the induction of anaesthesia the patient's teeth should be inspected. Laryngoscopy often imposes some strain on the teeth, and if they are abnormal, trauma is liable to result. Teeth may be pyorrhoeic and loose, or carious, or chipped; or fragile forms of dental prosthesis may be present. These more easily escape notice than subsequent injury. Porcelain inlays, bridgework, and single crowns screwed into the root of an incisor tooth are all very fragile.

In the past much stress has been laid upon preliminary medi-

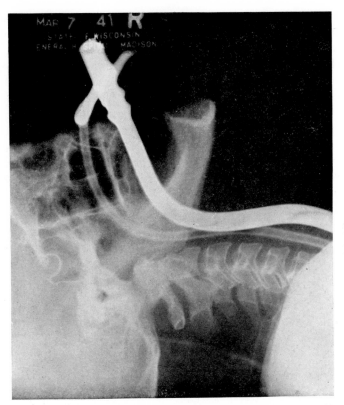

FIGURE 19.—LATERAL RADIOGRAPH OF THE HEAD AND NECK SHOWING ORAL
INTUBATION IN EDENTULOUS PATIENT WITH WOODBRIDGE TUBE

cation, and upon the anaesthetic agents and techniques used to procure anaesthesia. These considerations are entirely secondary to the main problem of securing ideal conditions for intubation, and their relation to intubation will be discussed later. Anaesthesia is progressively deepened until there is utter flaccid relaxation of the mandible and suppression of the pharyngeal and the glottic reflexes. When these conditions obtain, the beginner should deepen anaesthesia yet further, to be certain that they will persist during the time he requires to identify the structures and pass the tube. Laryngoscopy may then be undertaken.

Position.—The correct position of the patient upon the table materially facilitates the exposure of the larynx. Two alternative positions are recognized, the "classical" and the "amended." The classical position was described by Jackson[1] in 1913 as follows: "The patient's head must be in full extension, with the vertex firmly pushed down towards the feet of the patient, so as to throw the neck upward and bring the occiput down as close as possible beneath the cervical vertebrae." This position is shown diagrammatically in Figure 20. The shoulders lie flat on the table and the head is fully extended upon the neck. The drawback to this position is that it involves tension on all the muscles of the neck, and that the distance from the teeth to the glottis is increased. Nevertheless it furnishes very satisfactory exposure in many subjects.

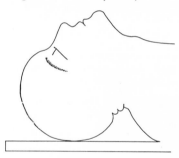 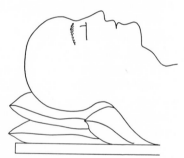

FIGURE 20.—THE "CLASSICAL" POSITION FOR LARYNGOSCOPY

FIGURE 21.—THE "AMENDED" POSITION FOR LARYNGOSCOPY

More recently Jackson has revised his earlier view[2] and suggested what is usually referred to as the "amended" position. The essential difference between this and the classical position is that while in both the scapulae remain flat on the table, in the amended position the head is raised at least ten centimetres above the level of the table, and is then slightly extended at the atlanto-occipital joint. In this position there is no tension on the muscles of the neck, and the distance from the teeth to the glottis is shortened. This position is shown in outline in Figure 21. Some workers have suggested the use of a gag to open the mouth before the insertion of the laryngoscope as a protection to the teeth.[3, 4] Jackson[1] has pointed out that to do this renders laryngoscopy more difficult because opening the mouth wide increases the tension on the muscles of the neck. If the induction of anaesthesia has been adequately carried out there should be relaxation of the mandible such as to render mechanical opening of the mouth superfluous. Nosworthy[5] and Magill[6] suggest that where patients have fragile teeth these can be protected from trauma by the use of adhesive strapping either on the blade of the laryngoscope or over the teeth, or both. Magill[7] originally used a piece of sheet lead for the purpose, but this is cumbersome.

Experienced and distinguished anaesthetists sometimes discuss with heat whether the right or the left hand should be used to insert the laryngoscope. Obviously if a right-handed worker wishes to use his right hand for both the manipulations involved in intubation, he must pass the laryngoscope with his right hand, and then hold it with his left hand while he passes the tube with his right. Equally obviously, anyone left-handed must either learn to pass the tube with his right hand or have a special laryngoscope made for his use with its channel in the left lateral position. It is a good plan for the beginner to hold the instrument with his fingers and not his palm. This makes it more difficult to apply force to the structures. If the induction of anaesthesia has been correctly carried out, the exposure of the larynx should be possible with a finger grip only. It is entirely immaterial how laryngoscopy is performed so long as it is atraumatic, efficient, and preferably rapid. The minor details of mechanical technique are best decided by the individual for himself.

Two methods of passing a laryngoscope are in common use: in the median line, and from the side of the mouth. For the beginner, who may have difficulty in identifying the structures, the median line makes recognition easy, but it involves passing the laryngoscope over the incisor teeth, which are more easily damaged than the molars. By the lateral route the laryngoscope is inserted at the right angle of the mouth and passed into the pharynx over the molar teeth, the tongue having been directed to the left side of the blade. When the instrument has a very wide channel and is not provided with a removable slide, or when it is passed in the median line, the tongue is liable to enter the lumen and obscure the view.

One hand inserts the laryngoscope into the mouth while the other separates the teeth to admit it, makes sure that the lips are not pinched between the blade and the teeth, and directs the tongue to the left of the spatula. The instrument is then slid along the dorsum of the tongue, past the uvula and the pillars of the fauces (frontispiece, 1), until the epiglottis comes into view (frontispiece, 2). Sise[8] has pointed out that smooth advancement of the laryngoscope in the pharynx is facilitated by pressure upon the end of the speculum with one thumb. The epiglottis is the chief landmark in laryngoscopy, inasmuch as it hangs down into the pharynx and conceals the glottic opening. The function of the laryngoscope is to lift up the epiglottis and so expose the glottis. This is done by advancing the laryngoscope a little further, until its beak lies beneath the epiglottis, and then lifting the instrument vertically upwards in the horizontal plane. No other exhibition of force is permissible during laryngoscopy, and this only if it is exercised in such a way that the pressure bears on soft tissues. Any tilting of the instrument, with the teeth as a fulcrum, must be avoided, because this movement is prone to damage both the teeth and the pharynx. As the epiglottis is lifted the glottis comes into view behind it (frontispiece, 3 and 4). The cords should be open. The false cords appear as red folds placed as the sides of an isosceles triangle, with the greyish true cords visible on their inner aspect. The trachea can often be seen extending down into the thorax. In cases in which the relaxation and the illumination are both good, the tracheal rings can be seen inside it, and sometimes even the carina can be made out. This view having been obtained, the lubricated tube is slipped through the open glottis into the trachea. If there is movement of the cords, the moment of greatest abduction should be chosen for intubation. The tube should be passed rapidly through the opening with one sweeping motion, care being taken to touch the cords as little as possible. Some authorities recommend that the tube be passed outside the barrel of the laryngoscope. When this is done, the view of the cords remains unobstructed and the tube approaches the glottis from behind and to the right. Others pass the tube directly down the speculum of the laryngoscope. The disadvantage of this technique is that a wide tube obstructs the view of the larynx, and the anaesthetist may be uncertain whether or not it has entered the trachea. The wider the tube, the less easy is its insertion, but when once the technique has been mastered the difference between wide and narrow tubes is scarcely noticeable. The mistake most commonly made by beginners is to pass the laryngoscope too far. The beak then lies in the cricoid sphincter of the oesophagus, which appears as a red puckered circle with a horizontal slit-like orifice in its centre and when the instrument is lifted the entire larynx is lifted with it and therefore not exposed to view. The solution is to withdraw the instrument until the epiglottis again appears, and then to pass the beak just under this structure and lift.

The above description of intubation sounds absurdly easy. Under the conditions which have been described it is as easy as it sounds. The beginner should therefore always make sure that these conditions obtain before embarking on laryngoscopy. If they are insisted upon, trauma is hardly possible.

Laryngoscopy and direct vision intubation can, however, be performed in various conditions of anaesthesia as well as in the conscious patient. Certain authors have described its performance with nitrous oxide[9, 10] and ethylene[11] anaesthesia, both of these being agents which, unless asphyxia to the verge of respiratory failure is super-added to anaesthesia, cannot produce the conditions described. The conditions of anaesthesia which normally obtain with these agents are the very opposite of those described above: the jaws are often tightly clenched, both pharyngeal and laryngeal reflexes are fully active, and the soft tissues are unrelaxed. Between these two extremes lie many conditions of anaesthesia in which intubation is rendered difficult by deficiencies both of relaxation and of reflex inhibition. These deficiencies are the chief cause of trauma, and trauma is the main disadvantage of intubation. On the other hand, the avoidance of trauma often involves a greater depth of anaesthesia than is necessary for the performance of the operation itself, and therefore an anaesthetist is constantly tempted to embark on laryngoscopy before he has secured adequate conditions for its performance. Increasing practice teaches that attempts to save two minutes usually result in the loss of fifteen, as well as the infliction of trauma. This much seems certain on this controversial point: that the beginner should incur none of these risks, even if the anaesthetist of mature skill may think himself justified in doing so in certain cases. As Hewer[12] says, " 'Safety first' as a slogan may be open to criticism for some purposes, but it is no bad motto for the anaesthetist."

Since the mask must be removed from the patient's face during laryngoscopy it follows that with each breath of air taken the anaesthesia is becoming lighter. To overcome this difficulty a few workers have suggested the pharyngeal insufflation of anaesthetic vapor during laryngoscopy.[13] If there is no longer adequate relaxation of the mandible by the time the laryngoscope is inserted, it may be difficult or impossible to expose the glottis. So much force is required to lift the epiglottis that trauma will probably be inflicted. Those skilled in laryngoscopy, however, do not need a complete exposure of the glottic slit to enable them to insert a tube. If the arytenoid cartilages can be seen, it follows that the glottis lies anteriorly to them. If any tube with a curve can be made to pass deeply anteriorly to the arytenoids, it must enter the glottis. The patient must not be allowed to recover to such an extent that he bites the laryngoscope, or trauma to the teeth becomes very likely.

The other chief trouble that results from imperfect conditions of anaesthesia is glottic spasm. If the glottic reflex has not been abolished, the stimulus of lifting the epiglottis with a laryngoscope will cause a spasm during which the false and true cords are tightly adducted (frontispiece, 6). In this state they cannot be passed with a rubber tube, and they may be seriously injured by forcing a passage with any rigid tube. This state of affairs can usually be avoided by producing a hyperpnoea by the use of carbon dioxide for a few moments before laryngoscopy is undertaken. If the carbon dioxide absorption technique is in use, the absorbent may be removed from the system for a few moments. If other methods are in use, a small quantity of carbon dioxide can be added to the mixture being respired by the patient.[6, 14] Glottic spasm can also be diminished by spraying the pharynx during inspiration with one of the local analgesic solutions (see page 63). This is recommended by many authorities. It can be done either before beginning the induction or before intubation. Probably the most efficient method is to expose the cords and then direct the spray at them through the laryngoscope.

When the tube has been inserted into the trachea it is firmly held in place by one hand while the other gently withdraws the laryngoscope, and fits between the teeth some form of "bite-block" to prevent the patient from biting the tube (see page 61). The tube should then be firmly secured to the lips or cheek of the patient by means of adhesive strapping. In spite of this precaution the anaesthetist should never loose his hold on the tube until the operation has actually begun and he is sure that there will be no further movement of the patient. In few hospitals as yet are the orderlies, surgeons, and assistants conscious of the fatal ease with which a tube can be pulled out of the trachea by a sudden unexpected movement of the patient or the apparatus.

TACTILE OROTRACHEAL INTUBATION

This technique demands the possession of long fingers by the anaesthetist. The author's experience is therefore limited to palpating the base of the tongue, and he can describe this technique only at second-hand! Deep anaesthesia, again with complete relaxation, abolition of reflexes, and hyperpnoea are desirable. The anaesthetist stands on a stool facing the patient at the right side of the table (if he is right-handed). The patient's mouth is opened wide and the tongue is drawn well out of the mouth by an assistant. The anaesthetist then passes his left index and medius along the dorsum of the tongue and feels for the epiglottis. This is hooked forwards by one finger while the other feels for the arytenoid cartilages. When these have been located, and the glottic opening has been palpated, the tube, which should be bent almost into a quarter circle by an intro-ducer, is passed along the guiding finger by the other hand, and so into the glottic opening. This was the technique used and described by Kühn (see Chapter I), and in recent years it has been revived by Sykes,[15] who feels that it is simpler and less traumatic than any method demanding laryngoscopy. He has therefore devised a modification of Kühn's tube. This has a rubber tip which enters the glottis and is passed with a curved introducer. The general opinion is, however, that tactile oral intubation is a method less certain of success than the visual technique, and one requiring more experience for its successful performance.

There are certain respiratory signs by which conviction may be acquired, after some experience, that the tube lies in the trachea and not in the oesophagus. These are considered under the heading of "blind nasal intubation."

BLIND OROTRACHEAL INTUBATION

This method was described by Troup[16] in 1935. He had found that if a Magill tube was passed through the mouth in the median line when the patient's head was in full extension, it would often enter the glottis without further instrumentation. In his view, intubation by this technique was facilitated by cutting the tube so that the point lay anteriorly instead of laterally when the tube was viewed from its concave aspect. In other respects his method resembled blind nasal intubation as de-scribed by Magill (see below, page 83). Troup's method was used tentatively in about a hundred cases by the anaesthetic staff of the London Hospital between the years 1936 and 1939.[17,18] Their method was to insert a "London Hospital Mouth Prop" (Figure 22) between the incisor teeth before in-duction, and to aim at anaesthesia providing full mandibular relaxation and hyperpnoea, though not necessarily complete abolition of the reflexes. When induction was complete the pil-

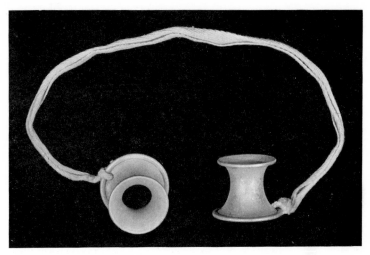

FIGURE 22.—LONDON HOSPITAL MOUTH PROP

low was removed, the head was placed in extreme extension on the neck, and the tube was passed through the mouth prop, the latter being used as though it were a nostril. These workers used the ordinary type of Magill tube with the bevel cut laterally. In their hands intubation by this technique proved successful in about sixty per cent of cases; in the remaining forty per cent laryngoscopy was necessary. Fortunately this technique most frequently succeeded in the type of patient in whom laryngoscopy usually presents difficulties: the large man with a short thick neck and a full set of teeth. It was found to be difficult in the aged and edentulous, for in these patients the tongue tended to fall back and obstruct the passage of the tube.

THE "DIVIDED AIRWAY"

This contrivance was put upon the market a few years ago in London, and no formal description either of it or of its use has appeared in the medical literature, although it is referred to by Challis[19] and Sykes.[15] It consists of a pharyngeal airway, circular in cross-section and made of a light metal, in two halves, which are held together by locking pins. Rubber tubes similar to Magill tubes are sold with it. They differ from the

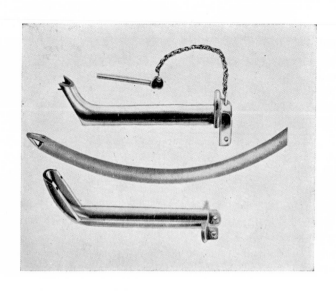

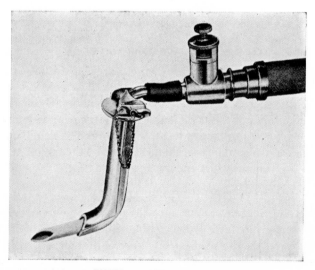

FIGURE 23.—DIVIDED AIRWAY

Above: Taken apart, showing fenestrated type of tube.
Below: Assembled, showing a Magill tube.

standard Magill tubes in that their tracheal end comes to a central point and is fenestrated (Figure 23). The airway is inserted when the pharyngeal reflexes have been abolished, and is used exactly like any other pharyngeal airway until the respiration is regular and automatic, with the cords opening well at each breath. Then the mask is removed and the tube is passed through the airway into the glottis. This technique of intubation is not successful in all cases, but it is probably as reliable as "blind" oral intubation. After the tube has been passed it is held in place by one hand while the other hand takes apart the two halves of the airway and withdraws them. The tube is connected to the anaesthetic supply in the usual way with an angle-piece. It is perhaps simpler to leave the airway in place around the tube during the operation, to prevent the tube from kinking or being bitten by the patient. Tubes of this type can be inserted by the blind nasal technique with no more difficulty than the standard pattern of Magill tube.[18]

THE INFLATABLE CUFF

As these cuffs are more commonly used by the oral route, it is appropriate to consider them at this point. The inflatable cuff is virtually the only means of ensuring a gas-tight endotracheal anaesthetic. The method is therefore of especial value whenever controlled respiration is to be used (see page 111) and whenever it is necessary to protect the respiratory tract from contamination by foreign fluids.

An endotracheal cuff should lie just below the vocal cords; if it lies more deeply in the trachea it is possible for foreign fluids to accumulate above it and to be aspirated into the respiratory tree when the cuff is deflated prior to extubation. Intubation is performed with the cuff in the completely deflated condition, and it is wise to defer its inflation until smooth anaesthesia has been re-established after the respiratory disturbances which usually accompany intubation have subsided. A dry syringe fitted with a blunt wide-gauge needle is then adapted to the inflating tube, and air is gently injected into the cuff. It is difficult for the inexperienced to gauge the degree of inflation

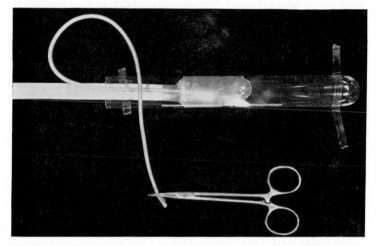

FIGURE 24.—LATERAL VIEW OF A CUFF DELIBERATELY OVER-INFLATED IN A GLASS
TUBE, SHOWING OBSTRUCTION AND COMPRESSION OF THE TUBE

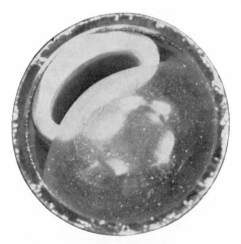

FIGURE 25.—TERMINAL VIEW OF THE OVER-
INFLATED CUFF, SHOWING COMPRESSION AND
OBSTRUCTION OF THE TUBE

required to assure a gas-tight fit without the use of excessive pressure. Originally Waters[20] recommended putting the cuff in a test-tube, where it could be seen, and practising its inflation to a suitable tension. Guedel[21] believes that several factors condition the pressure that should be used. The first of these is the size of the trachea, which has been found to increase with age, regardless of other factors.[14] The second is the length of the tracheal bearing surface of the cuff, and he believes that the optimum length is one and one-half inches. The third factor is the thickness of the wall of the cuff. Too thick a cuff will require so much pressure for its adequate inflation that a Magill tube may be collapsed by it. Too thin a cuff may bulge out in front of the tube (Figures 24 and 25) and so obstruct respiration. Guedel believes that over-inflation of the cuff may be responsible for trauma to the tracheal mucosa, and has suggested a practical test to ascertain the minimum necessary pressure. The breathing bag is held in one hand and the inflating syringe in the other. The cuff is then inflated until it just prevents the leakage of gases at the manual pressure on the bag required to cause expansion of the patient's chest. It has been found that since the thin rubber of the cuffs stretches with age, the actual quantity of air injected is an unreliable guide to effective inflation. If a cuff is over-inflated, a condition resembling a bronchial spasm is sometimes seen in which there is fixation of the chest and cyanosis.

Originally the cuffs were fitted on the tubes by covering the tube, the hands, and the cuff with French chalk, and then gradually "milking" the cuff on the tube with the fingers. Waters has recently devised a useful instrument to abolish the tedium of "milking" on the cuffs (Figure 26). Three metal rods rest in sockets in metal plates which can be spread apart by two handles working on the principle of a "chuck" on a lathe. The rods are placed inside the cuff and the handles of the instrument are approximated: this expands the cuff circumferentially, so the tube can be slipped inside it. The handles are then separated again and the metal rods withdrawn from the sockets in the plates and pulled from between the cuff and the

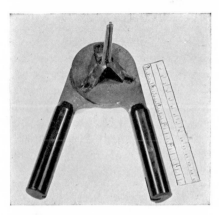

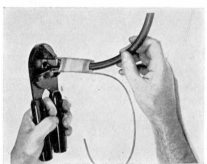

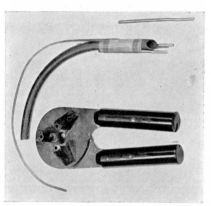

FIGURE 26.—INSTRUMENT FOR FITTING
INFLATABLE CUFFS

82

tube. The cuff should grip the tube firmly, so that it cannot slip over the end of the tube and obstruct respiration. A loose cuff may also slip off the tube at extubation and remain in the trachea. It is wise to test all cuffs before use by inflating them and immersing them in water.

NASOTRACHEAL INTUBATION

THE "BLIND" TECHNIQUE OF MAGILL[6, 7, 22, 23, 24, 25]

Nasal intubation is so frequently successful without recourse to laryngoscopy that when this route is to be used it is usually worth attempting the blind method before having recourse to laryngoscopy. It is futile for any worker to undertake a blind intubation unless he has had sufficient experience with direct vision intubation to be able to visualize the relative positions of the structures and their relationship to the unseen end of the tube. When for any reason the patient's mouth cannot be opened, the blind nasal method is the only way in which intubation is possible. It can be performed in almost any circumstances of anaesthesia in which there are audible breath sounds.

Magill recommends cocainization of the nose and pharynx before the induction of anaesthesia. Not only does this diminish the activity of the pharyngeal and laryngeal reflexes but it causes a shrinkage of the tissues in the nasal fossa and thus increases the space available for the passage of the tube and so lessens the likelihood of epistaxis. The nose should be examined beforehand in an attempt to determine which nostril offers least obstruction to the passage of the tube. The space available varies greatly in different persons. Edentulous patients, those whose nostrils appear to be flattened laterally, those with a history of nasal distortion, trauma, or operative interference, and children below the age of six are those in whom difficulties are usually encountered. Providentially enough, these are the very cases in which laryngoscopy is comparatively easy. Conversely, in the large plethoric man, who has a short thick neck and a full set of teeth, blind nasal intubation is usually easy.

It has already been pointed out that the degree of curve of a nasal tube has an important bearing on the ease with which blind intubation can be performed. This, however, is in relation to the position of the head of the patient when intubation is undertaken. The more curved the tube the greater the appropriate flexion of the head. Magill describes the ideal position of the

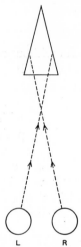
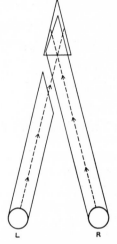

FIGURE 27A.—THE COURSE OF NASAL   FIGURE 27B.—THE MODUS OPERANDI OF
TUBES IN THE PHARYNX   THE BEVEL

head as that "of a man sniffing the air," and this position closely resembles the "amended" position for laryngoscopy (pages 70–71).

Magill tubes are sold cut in such a way that when looked at from the concave or anterior aspect the point is on the right and the bevel on the left (Figure 8). Magill noticed,[26] as MacEwen had in 1880 (page 8), that in normal individuals the courses of the nostrils tend to cross at a point in the oropharynx before reaching the glottis (Figure 27A). It was Magill's habit usually to attempt intubation through the right nostril, and it was his assumption that by cutting the tube to the shape described the bevel would meet the left vocal cord and the tube would be guided into the glottic opening (Figure 27B). Thus the standard Magill tubes are intended for use through the right nostril, and in his opinion blind intubation is easier with such a tube on that side. Several other workers feel that the "cut" of the tube makes little difference in the ease of intubation. For six years the author, in ignorance of Magill's view, has used the left nostril as a first choice in every case, and a standard Magill tube, and has found that the blind technique succeeded in ninety per cent of cases. Moreover, Troup[16] has suggested that nasal as well as oral intubation is facilitated by cutting the tube so that the point lies anteriorly instead of laterally.

Although blind intubation can be performed in any phase of anaesthesia from full consciousness to the fourth plane of the third stage, authorities disagree as to the influence of the plane of anaesthesia on the ease of intubation. Magill[6] feels that blind intubation is easiest before the onset of relaxation because the tonus of the muscles of the neck draws the epiglottis forward out of the line to the glottic opening. Other workers[23] have implied that complete muscular flaccidity facilitates blind intubation. It would seem that this varies with the patient. The easy case is not likely to be made easier by the presence of relaxation, whereas the difficult case may be, by reason of the greater mobility of the structures in this state. If, therefore, intubation is being performed in a subject requiring deep anaesthesia because of the nature of the operation, it is probably wise to defer any attempt at intubation until relaxation is present. On the other hand, if little relaxation is required for the operation, an early and successful attempt at blind intubation may spare the patient a superfluous degree of anaesthesia. Sometimes an induction which has been marred by pharyngeal obstruction or glottic spasm can be instantly "smoothed out" by a blind intubation. On the other hand, injudicious unsuccessful attempts at blind intubation increase the likelihood of minor trauma to the pharyngeal structures and often initiate a severe glottic spasm which previously did not exist. An attempt to save three minutes usually results in the loss of fifteen. No academic discussion of such points can carry the conviction to be derived from a few first-hand experiences. This much is certain: that the beginner should not attempt blind intubation in the absence of relaxation and the presence of the reflexes. In deep anaesthesia, if he fails to intubate by the blind technique, he can proceed at once to laryngoscopy and insert the tube without further trauma and loss of time. A sound "Gradus ad Parnassum" for the beginner in the technique of intubation is that he should master, in the following order, (1) laryngoscopic oral intubation in the fourth plane of the third stage; (2) nasotracheal intubation by direct vision in the fourth plane; (3) blind nasotracheal intubation in the fourth plane; and (4) blind nasal intubation in the first plane of the third stage, or in the second stage. Laryngoscopic intubation in light anaesthesia should be attempted only by workers with a great experience of intubation. "Open" tubes are easier of manipulation than those carrying cuffs, and semi-rigid tubes are easier to insert than flaccid ones. The beginner is wise who masters the easier methods before attempting the more difficult.

Blind Intubation in Deep Anaesthesia.—Anaesthesia is induced by any appropriate agents or techniques, the object being to secure complete relaxation, absence of all the reflexes, and hyperpnoea by the time intubation is to be attempted. The mask is then removed, and the tube, which has previously been lubricated, is passed through what the anaesthetist believes to be the freer nostril into the pharynx. De Caux [10] suggested lubricating the nostril rather than the tube, and it is possible that better results may be obtained in this way. Often the nares present some obstruction to the passage of the tube. It cannot be overemphasized that almost all epistaxis during nasotracheal intubation is due to the use of some force during the passage of the tube through the nose. This must be avoided. The tube is passed in its normal position: with the concavity lying anteriorly. If resistance is encountered in the nose the tube should be gently rotated in an effort to find a free passage. If this does not succeed, the tube should be withdrawn and the other naris explored. Sometimes—though fortunately rarely—both nares are impassable, and the anaesthetist must then choose between the abandonment of intubation, the use of orotracheal methods, or the careful use of pressure. Sometimes a narrower tube will pass without difficulty. Usually, however, patients are aware of serious degrees of nasal obstruction, and, if questioned beforehand, will put the anaesthetist on his guard. The course of the nasal fossa lies directly backward from the external nares (see Figure 28), following the line of the palate, and an effort should be made to induce the tube to follow this course. Figure 28 is the lateral radiograph of the head and neck of a healthy young adult in whom blind nasotracheal intubation had been performed. An opaque ureteric catheter was passed through the tube to make its course obvious. This radiograph clearly shows both the normal curve required in a nasal tube and the course of the nasal fossa.

It does not seem to be sufficiently realized that blind intubation depends almost entirely on the sense of hearing. As soon as the tube has passed from the nasopharynx to the oropharynx the anaesthetist should carefully note every sound to be heard

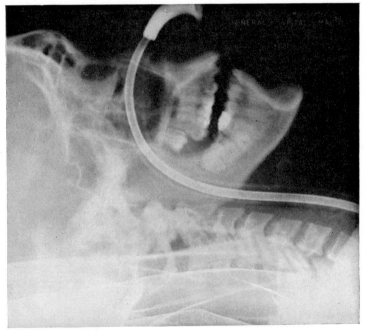

FIGURE 28.—RADIOGRAPH SHOWING A NASAL TUBE IN PLACE IN A NORMAL SUBJECT

through it. It follows that a quiet room for the induction of anaesthesia is highly to be desired for this reason alone; and that, conversely, the operating room proper is a difficult place in which to perform blind intubation. If the ear is kept close to the end of the tube the current of air can be felt as well as heard. The tube, once in the oropharynx, is advanced, the anaesthetist listening carefully to the character of the breath sounds heard through it. With his free hand he holds the head in extension at the atlanto-occipital joint in order to keep the epiglottis away from the posterior pharyngeal wall, and holds the opposite nostril closed to avoid confusion from the sounds of respiration through it. As long as the breath sounds increase in intensity the tube is following the proper course to the glottis and may be advanced. If the sounds diminish in intensity or disappear the tube is no longer advancing towards the glottic opening. In about fifty per cent of cases it will be found that the sounds increase in intensity until, at a certain point, the tube is felt in contact with the false cords and then glides farther in, the breath sounds losing their whistling character and acquiring a blowing quality. The changes in the nature of the breath sounds are characteristic and easily recognized after some experience. Only in very deep anaesthesia, however, will respiration continue to be regular after the insertion of a tracheal tube. In lighter planes the patient reflexly "holds his breath" for a few seconds. If the ear is kept close to the end of the tube a faint "panting" sound can often be heard during this "apnoea." This is probably due to the small amount of gaseous exchange promoted by the cardiac contractions, which can often be seen to cause a slight movement of a breathing bag during apnoea. If the anaesthesia has become light during the time taken to perform intubation, any of the phenomena described under "intubation in light anaesthesia" may be seen. To those sufficiently experienced to recognize them any of these respiratory phenomena are proof of successful intubation. Magill and others have laid stress on the technique of intubating during inspiration. It is natural to suppose that this is the most favorable time in the respiratory cycle; yet many tubes will enter the trachea during expiration, and the technique of passing a tube at the moment of an expulsive cough is well recognized (see page 94). If a tube is known to be of such a length as to reach from the nares to the middle of the trachea, and if respiration still takes place through it when it is fully inserted, its end must lie in the trachea and not in the oesophagus. This is the ultimate proof of successful blind intubation.

There are, obviously, four directions in which a tube may miss the glottic opening:

1. It may impinge upon the anterior commissure of the larynx, a condition usually due either to the use of too curved a tube or to excessive extension of the head. This position of the tube can be recognized by the fact that the maximum intensity of the sounds is succeeded, as the tube is advanced, by the acquisition of a high-pitched, whistling character. Then the tube is felt to encounter the resistance of the anterior commissure of the larynx, while the whistling sounds still persist. The remedy is to withdraw the tube slightly, increase the flexion of the head on the neck, and gently try again.

2. The course of the tube may be deflected posteriorly so that it enters the oesophagus. The tube advances easily to its full length, but the breath sounds are found to decrease and disappear after passing a point of maximum intensity. When the tube is in the oesophagus a very slight wet sucking sound, coincident with respiration, can often be detected by careful listening. This is due to the fact that the oesophagus usually contains some mucus and moves on respiration. Such a deviation of the tube from its true course results from the use of too straight a tube or excessive flexion of the head. The solution lies in further extension of the head. Figures 29, 30, and 31 show diagrammatically the mechanics of correction of antero-posterior deviations of a nasal tube. Figure 29 represents the position resulting from the use of too curved a tube or too much extension of the head. Figure 30 shows the correct alignment, with the tube in the trachea. In Figure 31 too straight a tube is in use or there is too much flexion of the head upon the neck; and the tube is in the oesophagus.

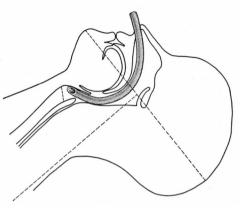

FIGURE 29.—EFFECT ON NASAL INTUBATION OF THE USE OF TOO CURVED A TUBE OR TOO MUCH EXTENSION OF THE HEAD

The tube is resting in the anterior commissure.

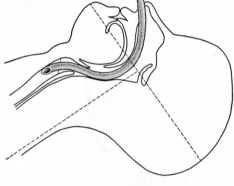

FIGURE 30.—THE CORRECT ALIGNMENT IN NASAL INTUBATION, SHOWING THE TUBE IN THE TRACHEA

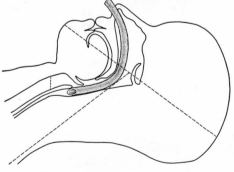

FIGURE 31.—EFFECT ON NASAL INTUBATION OF THE USE OF TOO STRAIGHT A TUBE OR TOO MUCH FLEXION OF THE HEAD

The tube is in the oesophagus.

3 and 4. Enlargement or displacement of the nasal septum or turbinates may cause deflections of the tube to right or left. In such cases it finds its way into one or other pyriform fossa, meets with a resistance to its advance, and the breath sounds previously heard through it vanish. Often the fingers of the left hand, resting on the skin of the neck, can feel the direction being taken by the tube; and sometimes the direction of the deflection can be seen from an obvious inclination to one side or the other of the tube in the nose. Two methods of overcoming lateral deflection are available. The first depends upon the fact that, owing to its curve, any rotation of the tube in the nose will cause its point to swing laterally in the pharynx. The tube therefore should be slightly withdrawn, rotated in the desired direction, and again advanced. The second depends upon the presence of sufficient relaxation of the soft tissues to enable the thyroid cartilage itself to be moved from side to side by the fingers of the left hand. This has been aptly described by Magill as "an attempt to thread the trachea on to the tube." The mechanism of the first method is shown diagrammatically in Figure 32.

In persons possessing a long epiglottis there is a tendency for a well-curved tube to find its way against the base of this structure (in the region known as the "vallecula") and be unable to advance. This position is shown in Figure 33. Holding

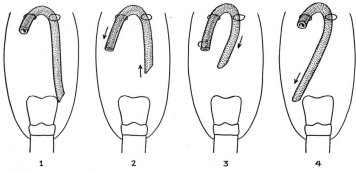

1   2   3   4

FIGURE 32.—EFFECT OF ROTATING THE NASAL END OF THE TUBE IN OVERCOMING
LATERAL DEFLECTIONS

the mandible well forward during the passage of the tube minimizes the incidence of this particular difficulty. If this artifice is unsuccessful the epiglottis can sometimes be circumvented by withdrawing the tube three inches, rotating it through ninety degrees, so that its end points laterally, and then inserting it again with a rotating movement so that it again re-

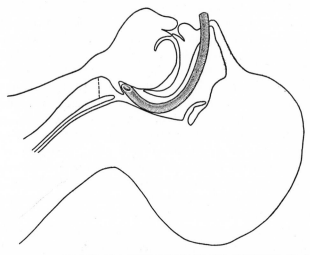

FIGURE 33.—POSITION OF A TUBE CAUGHT IN THE VALLECULA BY A
LONG EPIGLOTTIS

sumes its correct antero-posterior curve by the time it reaches the glottis. The rotatory movement involved is reminiscent of the technique of passing a large sound into the bladder. Naturally, if these various procedures fail, intubation by direct vision must be resorted to. Experience alone can teach when several attempts at blind intubation (which may often involve re-induction of anaesthesia) are justifiable because there is a likelihood of success and when they are not, and laryngoscopy should be undertaken forthwith. There is evidence to suggest that the incidence of respiratory complications after operation is increased by abortive attempts at blind intubation.[27] Probably the amount of manipulation is of less importance than the gentleness and smoothness with which it is carried out. Never should sufficient force be exerted to cause a Magill tube to kink in the pharynx: subtlety and not force is the key to blind intubation.

Blind Intubation in Light Anaesthesia.—Almost all the foregoing remarks apply equally to blind intubation deliberately undertaken in light anaesthesia. The conditions differ, however. Because of the character of the anaesthesia, the time available for intubation is short, and considerable skill is required to achieve rapid intubation without yielding to the temptation to use force in an attempt to save time. There is no relaxation of the jaw, which may be tightly clenched, and all the reflexes are fully active. Although "breath-holding" does not always preclude successful blind intubation, it renders it exceedingly difficult, and hyperpnoea is desirable if it can be obtained. The tube may go straight into the open glottis during either inspiration or expiration. If it does, there is usually a violent expulsive cough as the tube touches the tracheal mucosa, but the explosive character of the cough is lost because the cords can no longer close. Or the cords may close in adductor spasm as the tube touches them. If this happens, and the anaesthetist is sure that the point of the tube is resting on the glottic slit, he should simply wait, holding the tube gently in position on the closed cords. Two signs indicate such a position of the tube. The swallowing reflex is active under these conditions, and if the tube is resting on the glottis it will be seen to move up and down with the movements of deglutition. The cords are in spasm, and the characteristic high-pitched "squeal" of laryngeal spasm is unmistakable when heard at the proximal end of the tube. During this period of waiting "on closed cords" the patient may become slightly cyanotic. Quite suddenly, presumably when the accumulation of carbon dioxide reaches the level of the threshold to stimulus of the patient's respiratory centre, the patient either coughs or takes a very deep breath. If the tube is correctly placed it passes through as this occurs, and a violent cough usually accompanies its passage. Sometimes the movements of the larynx cause a tube which has already been placed in contact with it to slip off posteriorly into the oesophagus. This can often be overcome by an increase in extension of the head. Obviously a technique involving transitory oxygen deficiency must not be used in patients suffering from thyrotoxicosis, pulmonary lesions, or cardiac decompensation; nor must the state of hypoxia be allowed to persist for long. The pulse should be carefully observed during the period of waiting, for any irregularity of rhythm or undue slowing of rate suggests that the limit of the patient's tolerance is being approached. If intubation fails in light anaesthesia and re-induction to a deeper plane is practised, it often happens that a very easy blind intubation will result in the deeper plane. If the tube is left in the pharynx while this is done, provided it is neither kinked by the pressure of the mask nor in such a position as to irritate the glottis, it acts as a naso-pharyngeal airway, and the time necessary for the passage of the nose is saved when the second attempt is undertaken. If a tube is left in the nose while re-induction is performed, it sometimes happens that when the mask is removed the tube is found to have entered the glottic opening of its own accord during the re-anaesthetization.

It is unsafe to assume that if a patient is difficult to intubate by one method he will be equally difficult by another, as the following case illustrates:

A healthy man of thirty-five, weighing 190 pounds, was to have a submucous resection of the nasal septum. The nose had already been packed with gauze soaked in 20 per cent cocaine solution and adrenaline. Anaesthesia was induced by the nitrous oxide-oxygen-ether sequence, and laryngoscopy was attempted when complete relaxation of the mandible had been attained. The patient had an abnormally long and highly arched palate and a full set of teeth, and it was found impossible even to obtain a view of the arytenoid cartilages. Re-induction was undertaken as the anaesthesia became lighter, and on this occasion anaesthesia was deepened to the point of respiratory failure with ether and oxygen. Even in the presence of the utter flaccidity of all the structures then prevailing, neither the anaesthetist nor the aural surgeon was able to expose any portion of the glottis in any position of the patient. The packs were therefore removed from the nose. A No. 9 Magill tube, when inserted through the left nostril, passed directly, and at the first attempt, into a wide open glottis. The mouth was then opened wide, and while the fingers of one hand steadied the tracheal half of the tube in the pharynx, the nasal portion was hooked out of the nose through the mouth with the fingers of the other hand. The tube was then connected to the apparatus, the pharynx packed off with gauze, and the operation performed with smooth nitrous oxide–oxygen anaesthesia.

When difficulty in intubating is encountered by one route it is always wise to consider whether the alternative route might not yield better results.

NASOTRACHEAL INTUBATION BY DIRECT VISION

When blind nasal intubation fails, and nasotracheal anaesthesia is essential, laryngoscopy must be resorted to and the tube inserted into the trachea under direct vision. The technique of laryngoscopy is identical with that preceding oral intubation and requires no further discussion. When the glottic opening has been exposed to view the tube is passed through the nose and into the field of view of the laryngoscope. It is then almost always possible, by manipulating the tube, to cause it to enter the glottic opening. The experience of a few such visual nasal intubations is of great help to the beginner in making him realize the various deflections to which a nasal tube may be subject, and the movements which will correct for them. In a few cases where gross deformity of the structures exists it may be impossible to approximate the end of the tube to the glottic opening. It was for this contingency that the intubating forceps (Figure 15) was designed. It should not be used for the actual insertion of the tube into the glottis, least of all when the cords are in spasm. To attempt this is to court serious damage to the cords. The forceps should merely be used to place the tracheal end of the tube in such a position that gentle pressure on the nasal end will cause it to slide into the trachea. Cases requiring the use of forceps are rarely encountered by any anaesthetist who has mastered nasal intubation.

The most difficult type of case is that in which, when the glottis is exposed, the tube is found to be pointing anteriorly as it comes from the nose, whereas the trachea is leading posteriorly as well as downward; and the angle formed by the glottis between these lines (Figure 34) is acute. The author's

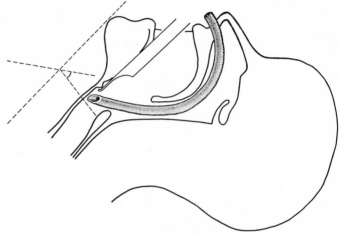

FIGURE 34.—DIAGRAM OF VISUAL NASAL INTUBATION ILLUSTRATING THE DIFFICULTIES TO WHICH TOO CURVED A TUBE MAY GIVE RISE

solution to this problem has been to place the point of the tube, by means of forceps if necessary, in the anterior commissure of the larynx, and then to withdraw the laryngoscope and lift the head into acute flexion on the neck. This movement causes the "angle" described to become more obtuse, and the tube usually slips in blindly at this point. This can be done whether the cords are active or open and flaccid.

Almost all visual nasal intubation can be achieved by slight alterations in the position of the tube or of the head or of the beak of the laryngoscope. Gentleness and subtlety are the secret of success.

INFLUENCE OF AGENTS ON EASE OF INTUBATION

THE "LIGHT" AGENTS: NITROUS OXIDE AND ETHYLENE

In the healthy adult patient neither of these agents can of itself produce the conditions of relaxation and reflex inhibition neces-

sary for atraumatic laryngoscopy without gross sub-oxygenation. If they are to be used for this purpose they must be preceded by a full basal narcosis, and cocainization of the larynx
is expedient. The experienced worker, however, can hope to
perform blind intubation successfully in about forty per cent
of cases without basal narcosis or sub-oxygenation. If basal narcosis is resorted to beforehand, blind intubation should succeed
in sixty or seventy per cent of cases.

In the very old or ill patient it is often possible to obtain
conditions permitting of laryngoscopy with one of these agents
alone. Lesions of the brain, especially those resulting in an increase in intracranial pressure, are wont to depress the glottic
reflex, and in patients suffering from these conditions intubation is correspondingly facilitated. The same is true of patients in extremis from surgical "shock" or asphyxia. This is
providential, for it enables any such patient, whose resuscitation demands a full and free supply of oxygen, to be intubated
with ease.

CYCLOPROPANE

Many anaesthetists feel that this is the ideal agent with
which to perform visual intubation. When the technique of
administration of the agent as well as that of intubation has
been mastered, this is probably true; for induction to a depth
of anaesthesia guaranteeing relaxation and reflex inhibition
is smoother and more rapid than with other agents. The beginner, however, is apt to administer a relative overdose during
induction, and so provoke an early depression of respiration
which makes it difficult to obtain deep anaesthesia. Cyclopropane anaesthesia is evanescent and therefore intubation must
be rapidly performed: there is no time for the beginner to
waste. On the other hand, cyclopropane is the most difficult
volatile agent with which to perform blind intubation. This
is partly due to the fact that the agent is not a respiratory stimulant, and partly to the fact that it is commonly administered by
the carbon dioxide absorption technique. The result is that the
respirations are so quiet as to be very difficult either to feel or
to hear.

DI-ETHYL ETHER

This is the most reliable agent with which to intubate, for it will provide all the above desiderata by whatever technique it is administered. Induction is more tedious than with cyclopropane, but the resultant anaesthesia lasts longer and more time is available for intubation. It is therefore the best agent for the use of the beginner while he is learning to intubate. As it is a respiratory stimulant it gives rise to conditions under which blind intubation is at its easiest.

CHLOROFORM

Whatever doubts may have existed as to the practicability of endotracheal chloroform anaesthesia in the early days of insufflation (see pp. 40–41), the experience of the past fifteen years in England has clearly shown that these are ill founded when applied to modern conditions. Nowadays chloroform is chiefly used as an adjuvant to nitrous oxide, and when it is so used the danger of overdose, the possibility of chemical damage to the tracheal mucosa, and the likelihood of toxic hepatitis in the postoperative period are all minimized. The conditions necessary to atraumatic visual intubation can be realized with certainty with this agent. For purposes of blind intubation chloroform is satisfactory, but because it is a respiratory depressant it produces less easy conditions than does ether. The beginner is apt to find blind intubation with chloroform difficult, but experienced workers are not unduly inconvenienced. Whenever intubation is desirable in the presence of a fire hazard, chloroform, either alone or as an adjuvant to mixtures of nitrous oxide and oxygen, deserves careful consideration.

THE INTRAVENOUS BARBITURATES

The two ultra-short-acting substances known as "Evipal" and "Pentothal" have but a narrow margin of dosage separating reflex inhibition from respiratory failure. Both, especially the former, appear to increase the reflex irritability of the glottis, and if the cords develop adductor spasm it is usually severe. Efficient local analgesia of the glottis can overcome the latter difficulty. The former remains. Muscular relaxation may be difficult to obtain in robust patients, but is usually complete in old, young, or debilitated subjects. Therefore, while it may be legitimate for experienced workers to incur the risks attendant upon intubation after an induction with an intravenous barbiturate, this technique should not be attempted by the novice. Blind intubation can be performed by the expert, but is rendered extremely difficult by the respiratory depression these substances produce, as well as by the increased irritability of the glottis.

AVERTIN

This substance also depresses respiration, although not so sharply as do the intravenous barbiturates. It also depresses the irritability of the glottic reflex, but full muscular relaxation is rarely seen. Thus laryngoscopy is usually difficult after induction with avertin, and blind intubation fairly difficult because of the respiratory depression. The use of nitrous oxide following basal narcosis with a non-volatile agent will often stimulate respiration and so produce conditions in which intubation is relatively easy. Momentary relaxation, sufficient for rapid laryngoscopy, can usually be obtained; and the stimulant effect of the nitrous oxide upon the respiration increases the likelihood of successful blind intubation.

THE INFLUENCE OF TECHNIQUE

The various techniques by which anaesthetics may be administered do not greatly influence the ease of intubation. The extent to which any technique of anaesthesia helps or hinders intubation is largely a matter of the degree to which it causes an accumulation of carbon dioxide. This substance causes hyperpnoea, and thus promotes a rapid induction of anaesthesia and an early onset of the conditions which facilitate intubation. When using an open technique there is no accumulation of carbon dioxide until respiratory depression occurs in deep anaesthesia. The semiclosed technique leads to some accumulation of carbon dioxide, and hyperpnoea is usually manifest in the first few minutes. Most machines designed for this work are equipped with facilities for adding even more carbon dioxide to the inspired vapor. The carbon dioxide absorption technique, while it gives rise to a higher concentration of carbon dioxide beneath the mask than is present in the inspired air, prevents an increase in this concentration. There results an amplitude of respiration resembling that of the normal sleeping individual. It follows that the time necessary for induction to deep anaesthesia with this technique is much longer than when carbon dioxide is allowed to accumulate. Whatever technique of induction is used, it is generally conceded[14] that the use of an increased concentration of carbon dioxide is legitimate for a few moments before intubation. If the absorption technique is in use the absorbent may be removed from the system in an effort to produce hyperpnoea. The abuse of carbon dioxide is as dangerous as its judicious use is convenient. As soon as intubation has been performed the anaesthetist should satisfy himself that the efficient elimination of carbon dioxide has again been ensured.

One of the objections to intubation raised by surgeons is the additional time consumed during induction. An experienced worker should be able to intubate any but the most difficult patients in ten minutes from the time of application of the mask. The beginner will often require thirty minutes.

Since blind intubation depends entirely upon the ability of the anaesthetist to discover and follow the direction of the breath sounds, it follows that hyperpnoea facilitates this manoeuvre. For this reason cyclopropane anaesthesia—indeed all anaesthesia by the absorption technique—and the practice of blind intubation are mutually inimical. This fact probably explains the hesitancy with which England has adopted the absorption technique, and the United States the practice of blind intubation.

EXTUBATION

Three complications may occur when an endotracheal tube is removed, and these must be foreseen and prevented. They are trauma, respiratory obstruction, and the aspiration into the trachea of foreign fluids or substances.

Opinions differ as to the likelihood of inflicting trauma during extubation. Some workers prefer to leave a tube in place until the patient regains consciousness rather than risk respiratory obstruction. Others feel that this course is conducive to the incidence of tracheitis or laryngitis in the postoperative period. Flagg[28] recommends re-anaesthetization to deep anaesthesia if the cords are felt to grip the tube. This is a wise precaution if a metal tube is used, but is superfluous with smooth rubber or semi-rigid tubes.

Respiratory obstruction may result from spasm of the glottis when the tube is removed. If the patient is deeply anaesthetized when extubation is performed, the glottic reflex will be inactive and spasm will not occur. Many workers also believe that spasm will not occur in light second-stage anaesthesia, but this is a controversial point. If a tube is removed in any plane between the middle of the second stage and the lower border of the second plane of the third stage, glottic spasm may occur, and is often severe if ether is in use. Provided the patient's airway is otherwise patent the worst that will occur is a transitory cyanosis, but if pharyngeal obstruction is permitted as well, a serious oxygen deficiency will result. Very gentle and gradual removal of the tube from the glottis minimizes the incidence and severity of the spasm. If any pharyngeal obstruction is present after extubation a pharyngeal airway should be inserted; and this precaution should also be observed whenever extubation is performed in deep anaesthesia. The anaesthetist should never leave a patient after extubation until he is satisfied that unobstructed normal respiration has been re-established.

Blood, mucus, or operative disjecta may accumulate in the pharynx during endotracheal anaesthesia. These must be removed by suction or by swabbing out the pharynx before the tube is removed, lest they be aspirated into the respiratory tract. Cases have occurred in which the anaesthetist failed to remove a pharyngeal pack at the end of an operation, or where the mouth prop was allowed to fall into the pharynx. If the patient is lightly anaesthetized and the pharyngeal reflexes are active, a foreign body will probably be expelled. If, however, the reflexes are absent this will not occur, and severe respiratory obstruction will probably result. Cuffed tubes should be removed by simultaneous traction upon the tube and the inflating tube, lest the cuff be pulled off the tube and remain in the trachea. If a tube is left in place until the patient recovers consciousness the anaesthetist must be certain that it is duly removed. One case has occurred in which, the angle-piece having become detached, a Magill nasal tube was aspirated into the tracheo-bronchial tree, where it gave rise to the signs of a pulmonary abscess before being coughed out by the patient on the fourth day after operation.

Patients in whom a fractured jaw has been reduced, a spinal graft has been performed, or a torticollis has been corrected are often placed, during anaesthesia, in positions conducive to respiratory obstruction, the maintenance of which is ensured by traction or plaster casts. If these patients have been intubated the greatest care must be taken to ensure a free airway when the tube is removed. Anaesthesia should be as light as possible at the close of the operation, and the anaesthetist should not leave the patient until he is satisfied that no obstruction exists. Similar precautions are wise in nose and throat cases in which the upper respiratory passages are usually obstructed by blood.

REFERENCES

1. JACKSON, C. Surg. Gyn. & Obs. 1913. XVII. 507.
2. ————Bronchoscopy, Oesophagoscopy, & Gastroscopy. 3d ed. Philadelphia, 1934. pp. 85-91.
3. FLAGG, P. J. Arch. Otolaryngol. 1932. XV. 844.
4. HARGRAVE, R. C. M. A. J. 1934. XXX. 633.
5. NOSWORTHY, M. D. The Theory and Practice of Anaesthesia. 1st ed. London, 1935. p. 131.
6. MAGILL, I. W. Am. Jour. Surg. 1936. XXXIV. 450.
7. ————Curr. Res. Anaes. & Analg. 1931. X. 164.
8. SISE, L. F. Surg. Clinics N. America, 1934. XIV. 1049.
9. STEWART, C. C. Curr. Res. Anaes. & Analg. 1933. XII. 49.
10. DE CAUX, F. P. Brit. Jour. Anaes. 1931. IX. 22.
11. GRIFFITH, H. R. C. M. A. J. 1929. XXI. 294.
12. HEWER, C. L. Recent Advances in Anaesthesia & Analgesia. Preface to first edition. London, 1932.
13. KAVANAGH, M. Calif. State Jour. Med. 1922. XX. 425.
14. GUEDEL, A. E. & WATERS, R. M. Ann. Otol. Rhinol. & Laryngol. 1931. XL. 1139.

15. Sykes, W. S.   Curr. Res. Anaes. & Analg. 1937. XVI. 133.
16. Troup, G.   Curr. Res. Anaes. & Analg. 1935. XIV. 249.
17. Challis, J. H. T.   Personal Communication. 1938.
18. Gillespie, N. A.   Unpublished Data.
19. Challis, J. H. T.   Curr. Res. Anaes. & Analg. 1937. XVI. 82.
20. Gale, J. W. & Waters, R. M.   Curr. Res. Anaes. & Analg. 1932. XI. 283.
21. Guedel, A. E.   Personal Communication. 1941.
22. Magill, I. W.   Newcastle Med. Jour. 1934. XIV. 67.
23. Lewis, I. N.   Brit. Med. Jour. 1937. II. 630.
24. Magill, I. W.   Brit. Med. Jour. 1930. II. 817.
25. ————Proc. Roy. Soc. Med. (Anaes.) 1928. XXII. 83.
26. ————Personal Communication. 1940.
27. Dawkins, C. J. M.   Brit. Jour. Anaes. 1937. XIV. 182.
28. Flagg, P. J.   The Art of Anaesthesia. 6th ed. Philadelphia, 1939. p. 378.

VI. MISCELLANEOUS TECHNICAL CONSIDERATIONS DURING MAINTENANCE

THE APPROPRIATE LENGTH AND BORE OF
ENDOTRACHEAL TUBES

IT WAS CUSTOMARY in the early days of endotracheal anaesthesia to regard the bifurcation of the trachea as lying twenty-six centimetres from the incisor teeth.[1] Individuals vary so greatly in size that no measurements can ensure a correct length of tube, and this fact was soon realized by anaesthetists. The point is of less importance in inhalation endotracheal anaesthesia, in which the end of the tube may lie anywhere between the larynx and the bifurcation, than in insufflation, where it is necessary that the tip lie at the bifurcation itself. The length of inhalation tubes can be adequately measured by laying them alongside the patient's neck. The trachea bifurcates at the level of the "Angle of Louis"—that of the second costal cartilage—and it begins at the lower border of the cricoid cartilage. Any inhalation tube whose end lies between these two points is of the proper length, and this leaves a "margin of error" of at least nine centimetres. Naturally this length must be measured either from the incisor teeth or the nares according as the route of intubation is the oral or the nasal. If a tube is too long it will usually enter the right main bronchus, and the bevel of a Magill tube then meets the medial wall of the bronchus and the tube becomes completely obstructed. Figure 35 shows the radiographs of the chest of a patient in whose case this error was committed. Forty-five minutes after intubation it was observed that there was diminished movement of the left side of the chest. The radiograph at the left was taken at that point. The tube was then withdrawn one inch, the anaesthesia was lightened, and the patient was encouraged to cough. Anaesthesia was then deepened again and the chest was inflated gently twice from the breathing bag. The radiograph at the right in Figure 35 was then taken; and it shows that the lungs had already been almost

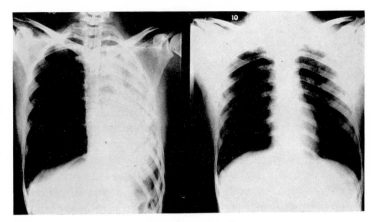

FIGURE 35.—RADIOGRAPHS OF THE CHEST OF A PATIENT WHOSE RIGHT MAIN
BRONCHUS HAD BEEN INTUBATED BY MISTAKE

completely re-expanded. The right main bronchus is more
usually entered than the left because its course is straighter;
the left main bronchus makes a more acute angle with the
trachea. Fatalities have resulted from the inadvertent intubation
of a main bronchus where the anaesthetist was not alive to the
possibility and failed to notice an abnormality of respiration. If,
after intubation, the patient continues to cough after a few
breaths of the anaesthetic vapor and shows a disinclination to
"settle down" into smooth anaesthesia, especially if there be
cyanosis and asymmetrical movement of the chest, inadvertent
intubation of a bronchus has probably occurred, and the tube
should be withdrawn an inch or so. The mistake is most commonly made in small infants who tolerate such an interference
with respiration badly.

The diameter of tube to be used in any given patient is a
vexed question. It is difficult to compare the circular bore of a
round tube with that of a triangular orifice such as the glottis.
Tuffier[2] stated that in the average adult the glottic opening is
an isosceles triangle whose sides measure 25 millimetres and
whose base is 8 millimetres wide. The area of such a triangle
is 98 square millimetres. Since the areas of Nos. 10, 9, and 8

Magill tubes are respectively 113, 94, and 80 square millimetres, it seems reasonable to suppose that in the average adult the glottic opening is slightly increased by the passage of a 13-millimetre tube, but unchanged by any smaller size. In practice it is as easy for the hypercritical to imagine obstruction where none exists as for the indolent to overlook its obvious signs. The recent tendency has been to become more conscious of minor degrees of obstruction, and therefore the tubes in use grow ever wider. So far the maximum reached is about 14 millimetres in diameter. Probably the technique used to supply anaesthetic vapor to the patient plays some role in determining the size of tube necessary to minimize respiratory obstruction; for obviously the placing of any tube in the glottis must restrict its lumen to some extent unless the tube is so wide as to cause an abduction of the cords greater than normal. When a tube is used as a "laryngeal airway" under a mask, such a restriction occurs, but if the glottis is not in spasm gaseous exchange can take place around as well as through the tube. When the tube is connected directly to the source of vapor this is supplied to the tube at a very slight positive pressure, and probably this pressure compensates, by a slight degree of insufflation, for any restriction of the glottic orifice. When the tube is "closed off" by an inflatable cuff or packing, the patient is forced to achieve all his gaseous exchange through the tube in both directions; and under these conditions respiration may become labored if too small a tube is used. In practice it will be found that all adult requirements can be met by the use of tubes of the Magill sizes 6 to 9, and even these are wider than the nine-millimetre tube which, even with the amount of dead space allowed by Kühn (see page 14) did not apparently give rise to serious accidents. Deficient oxygenation is seldom seen in a patient who has been intubated, and when it does occur it is more usually due to a depression of respiratory movement than to any narrowing of the airway by the tube. It is important that rubber tubes for nasal use should have walls as thin as possible to minimize the restriction of airway, for smaller tubes must be used through the nose than can be passed through the mouth. The manufacturers have attempted to meet this difficulty by marketing thin-walled Magill tubes marked "nasal" and thick-walled ones marked "oral." The activity of respiration also influences the size of tube necessary to free breathing. Other things being equal, the greater the minute-volume of respiration, the larger will be the tube required to avoid signs of obstruction.

THE EFFECT OF INTUBATION ON THE DEAD SPACE

Since gaseous exchange does not take place in the dead space of the respiratory tree, it follows that any modification of the volume of the dead space will enhance or diminish the efficiency of respiration. Guedel and Waters[3] have measured the cubic content of the mouth, nose, and pharynx of the anaesthetized patient, and have found it to vary between 60 and 75 cubic centimetres. If the cubic content of Magill tubes is measured by clamping the tube at the point at which the glottis usually rests and filling it with fluid, it is found that the content of a No. 10 tube is 14 cubic centimetres, that of a No. 9 is 11 cubic centimetres, and that of a No. 7 is 9 cubic centimetres. From these facts it seems that intubation reduces the dead space by about 50 cubic centimetres and therefore enhances the efficiency of respiratory exchange. When the tube is connected directly to the source of vapor, the dead space is further diminished by about 150 cubic centimetres, which is the approximate content of most masks. This conclusion is supported by the apparent increase in efficiency of even minimal respiratory movements in the intubated patient.

METHODS OF MAINTENANCE

During any operation whose performance is not hindered by the presence of a mask upon the face an endotracheal tube may be used as a "laryngeal airway," the mask being replaced on the face after the tube has been passed. Adhesive strapping, safety pins passed through the tube, rubber flanges cemented on the proximal end of the tube, and "funnel" type angle-pieces are all commonly used to ensure that the tube does not slip into the pharynx through the mouth or nose. When the use of a face-

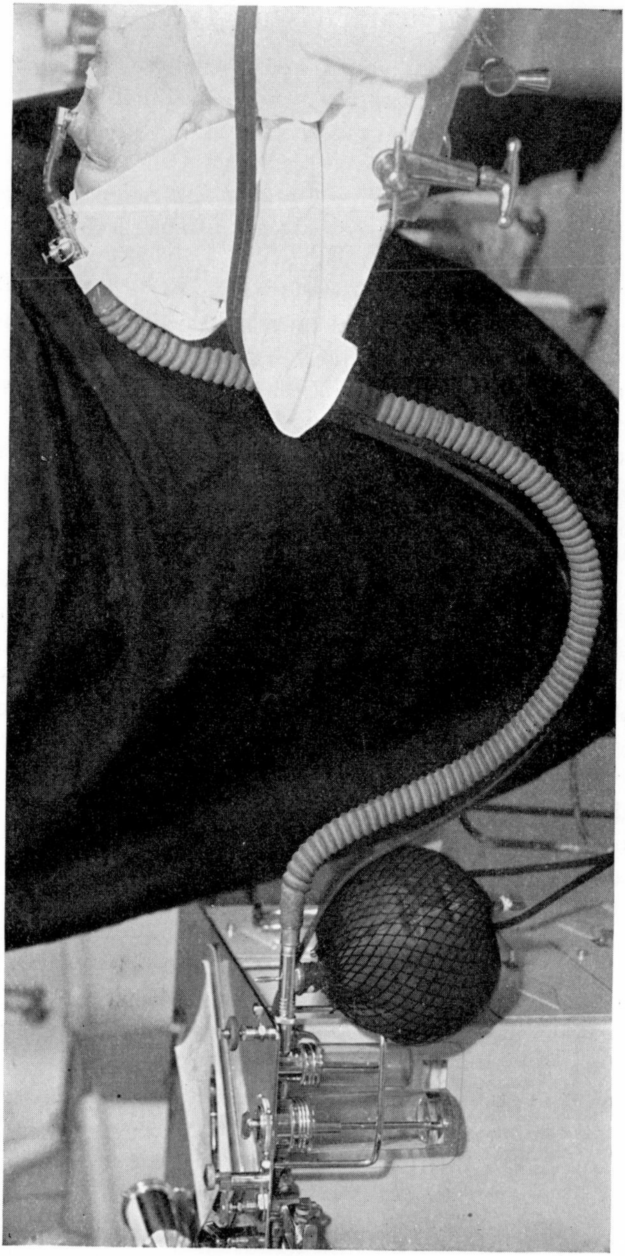

FIGURE 36.— "MAGILL'S ATTACHMENT" IN USE

piece is undesirable the tube is connected directly to the source of vapor by means of a short piece of rubber tubing and a metal adaptor. The methods of maintenance fall into four broad categories:

"Primitive" Methods.—The simplest and oldest of these consists of the use of a gauze-covered funnel attached to the tube by a piece of rubber tubing, which should be as short as possible. The anaesthetist drops the agent on the gauze, holding the funnel below the level of the larynx to make sure that none of the liquid enters the lungs. Flagg's "tin can" method,[4] whereby the patient is allowed to breathe air which has passed over the surface of liquid ether, is a modification of this. Both methods, however, involve a considerable increase in the respiratory dead space. An endotracheal tube can of course be used as a laryngeal airway under an open gauze mask.

"Semiclosed" Methods.—The endotracheal tube is connected to the breathing tube of the machine by means of an adaptor. At the machine end of the breathing tube is a thin rubber bag. As close to the face as possible there is a spring-loaded expiratory valve, which is so lightly adjusted as to blow off at a pressure of one millimetre of mercury. This arrangement of apparatus is shown in Figure 36. The gases are kept constantly flowing through this system at a rate of not less than five litres a minute. When the bag is full the valve opens and any excess of gas escapes. This occurs at the end of each expiration, and thus that part of expiration containing the highest concentration of carbon dioxide is eliminated. The high rate of flow of the gases is necessary to ensure this elimination. If an increase in intrapulmonic pressure is desired, it can be obtained by increasing the tension at which the expiratory valve opens. In certain types of apparatus the breathing bag is incorporated in the machine; the "Magill's attachment" shown in Figure 36 is commonly used in Great Britain for the purpose. The method is uneconomical, for large quantities of anaesthetic agents must of necessity be wasted in order to eliminate excess carbon dioxide. Only one breathing tube is necessary to this technique, and a minimum of heavy apparatus directly attached to the

endotracheal tube. Kinking and displacement of the tube during operations on the head are therefore less frequently a source of trouble when this method is in use. When an endotracheal tube without a cuff or pharyngeal pack is in place, a slight tightening of the expiratory valve causes a small quantity of the gases to leak out between the tube and the tracheal walls. This is really inhalation with some degree of insufflation.

The To and Fro Absorption System.—The tube is connected by an adaptor to a canister which contains soda-lime and which has a breathing bag attached to its outer end. The connecting tube should be as short as possible so that the dead space is not unduly increased. Of necessity the canister must remain close to the head, and this fact renders the to and fro system an inconvenient method in operations upon the head, because the weight of the canister is apt to displace or kink the tube. It has the advantage, however, that the breathing bag is close to the anaesthetist's hand. This enables manual alterations of the volume of respiration to be carried out easily, and is useful in operations conducted with "controlled" respiration (see page 111).

The "Circle" Absorption System.—Two breathing tubes, provided with valves forcing the respiratory gases to circulate in one direction only, are necessary. These are connected to the endotracheal tube by means of a T- or Y-piece and a short piece of rubber tubing. King[5] has recently suggested an adaptor which will overcome many of the difficulties associated with the convenient fixation of the tubes of a circle filter in operations upon the head. Both the breathing bag and the canister are accommodated on the anaesthetic machine, and there is therefore less weight which may cause displacement or kinking of the tube. The bag is usually at a distance from the head, and therefore the manual control of respiration is less easy than with the to and fro system.

If any of the absorption methods are used without an inflatable cuff or a pharyngeal pack, much higher flows of the gases are usually necessary because of the leakage of gases which occurs between the tube and the glottis. They thus become a mixture of inhalation and insufflation anaesthesia, the bag being kept full in complete expiration by running into the system a sufficient excess of vapor to compensate for the loss by leakage.

CONTROLLED RESPIRATION

In 1934 it was suggested by Guedel and Treweek[6] that apnoea could be produced in the course of anaesthesia at will, where the carbon dioxide absorption technique was in use, by a manual augmentation of respiratory exchange through the absorbent, and an increase in the ether concentration. During such an apnoea voluntary respiratory movements are absent and their function is assumed by the anaesthetist, who can then regulate ventilation at will. At that time Woodbridge suggested the name "passive" respiration to describe this variety of apnoea. In 1936 Waters[7] described his use of this technique under the title of "controlled" respiration, and Nosworthy[8] has recently discussed its utility in thoracic operations. It has been extensively used in the last five years, and has proved of service in interventions in the thorax and the abdomen where an intermittently motionless field of operation is desirable. The freedom of airway assured by intubation, although not essential to the use of controlled respiration, facilitates its performance.

When it is desired to establish controlled respiration, the anaesthetist augments the volume of exchange by manual pressure upon the breathing bag during inspiration, releasing his hold promptly during expiration to encourage emptying of the lungs. When exchange has thus been augmented during several inspirations it is found that if pressure on the bag is then omitted, no further respiratory movement takes place. The anaesthetist then maintains respiratory exchange by manual pressure on the bag; and he should strive to reproduce the rate and volume of exchange in the normal sleeping individual. In those operations in which a motionless field is of assistance to the surgeon the anaesthetist stands holding the breathing bag lightly and watching the surgeon's movements. As soon as the latter turns from his field to pick up an instrument, or otherwise interrupts his work, the lungs are gently inflated from the bag. Between these inflations the field of operation remains still.

A leakproof endotracheal technique, such as is provided by the use of an inflatable cuff, is the ideal when controlled respiration is to be used. Otherwise there is a loss of anaesthetic vapor at each compression of the bag, and it may become difficult to maintain anaesthesia at a constant level. This object may also be attained by using an endotracheal tube under the anaesthetic mask, but if this is done some of the vapor may be forced into the stomach by the pressure on the bag.

The institution of controlled respiration should not be undertaken until the depth of anaesthesia is such that the tracheal reflex is abolished and the presence of the tube no longer causes reflex "breath-holding." So long as the patient is coughing or holding his breath the intercostal muscles are contracted, and inflation of the lungs can be achieved only by the exertion of considerable pressure, which may be dangerous.

THE RELATION OF ENDOTRACHEAL ANAESTHESIA TO INTRABRONCHIAL AND INTRATHORACIC PRESSURE

A patient who has not been intubated can close his glottis and so protect his air passages to some extent from the effects of positive pressure applied to the breathing bag. When a tube is in place in the trachea any positive pressure at which the gases are supplied will raise the intrabronchial pressure. Whenever the trachea is intubated the anaesthetist must strive to avoid the imposition of positive pressure on the respiratory tree. When semiclosed methods are in use the expiratory valve should be set to blow off at a very low positive pressure, for this will protect the patient in any eventuality. When completely closed systems are in use, especially if a cuff or pack is used to preclude the leakage of gases at the glottis, it is important that the breathing bag be not completely filled, for a loose bag makes the imposition of positive pressure unlikely.

There are occasions, however, on which the use of some positive pressure is both necessary and justifiable. When one or both pleural cavities are opened the use of positive pressure is essential to prevent collapse of the lung. When the thorax is to be closed again it is desirable that the lung be fully distended at the moment of closure, so that as little air as possible is left in the pleural cavity. It has been known since the days of Tuffier[9] that a pressure of ten centimetres of water (or six millimetres of mercury) is sufficient to maintain distension of the lungs in the presence of pneumothorax. A similar pressure, intermittently applied, suffices for the institution of controlled respiration. The application of intermittent pressure coincident with the normal cycle of respiration is probably less disturbing both to respiration and to circulation than the maintenance of a constant positive pressure during both phases of respiration. Pulmonary oedema is sometimes seen during anaesthesia, and it may be, as Barach[10] suggests, that the use of a positive pressure in the region of four millimetres of mercury will help to counteract the establishment of this condition. Experimental work recently published by members of the staff of the University of Chicago Clinics[11, 12, 13] suggests that caution should be exercised in the use of positive pressure, for there are two distinct ways in which it may be harmful.

The first of these is the direct effect of pressure upon the lungs themselves. In 1917 Georg[14] demonstrated the occurrence of emphysema in dogs after the use of insufflation pressures of twenty-five to thirty millimetres of mercury. Marcotte *et al.*[11] have recently found that an intrabronchial pressure of twenty-four millimetres of mercury usually produced mediastinal emphysema in dogs, and have seen it occur at eighteen millimetres. In cats the lower pressures of sixteen to twenty millimetres of mercury were sufficient to produce emphysema. Heidrick *et al.*[13] have reported a case in which the use of a pressure of twelve millimetres to distend the lung during closure of the thorax in the human subject was followed by emphysema. Bradshaw[15] has recently reported a case in which a proposed thoracic operation in an infant was abandoned because of the appearance of emphysema following intubation. As he mentioned no details of the technique used, one can only speculate as to the cause. The experimental work of Macklin[16, 17] has demonstrated, by the use of very high intrabronchial pressures in experimental animals, exactly how such an emphysema occurs. He showed that air could break through in small bubbles from over-distended alveoli to the peri-vascular connective tissue, and could track along the course of the arterioles to the great vessels. Marcotte *et al.*[11] are of the opinion that this process can take place more easily when the thorax is open. Similar results have been reported in the human being subjected to high intrapulmonic pressures,[18] and there is little doubt that this concept of the production of emphysema is correct.

The other reasons for which the use of positive pressure should be avoided are physiological. For many years it has been recognized that the efficiency of the circulation is handicapped by an increase in intrathoracic pressure. In any intubated subject whose thorax is intact an increase in intrabronchial pressure will of necessity increase the intrathoracic pressure. This means that a back pressure is set up which hinders the return of blood through the Vena Cava and therefore the filling of the right auricle; and the output of the heart falls in consequence. Eisenbrey[19] and Janeway[20] pointed out these facts in the early days of endotracheal anaesthesia. Marcotte *et al.* have demonstrated a fall in blood pressure in every animal in which they have raised the intrabronchial pressure, the first varying almost directly as the second. A practical demonstration of this fact can often be seen during anaesthesia, for an increase in the pressure at which vapor is administered to the patient causes a venous and capillary engorgement which inconveniences the surgeon by increasing capillary haemorrhage, and which will subside at once when the pressure is reduced.

Intrabronchial pressures during endotracheal anaesthesia depend upon the relation between the pressure at which vapor is admitted to the tube and the pressure at which it can escape from the trachea. These pressures are influenced by the type of apparatus in use, and the extent to which the escape of gases between the tube and the respiratory passages can occur.

Thus if suction is applied to one tube passed into the trachea, and the cords close around the tube, an application of negative pressure to the alveoli will result. This may cause an atelectasis, and Barach[21] feels that it is conducive to the incidence of pulmonary oedema. On the other hand, if gases are insufflated into the bronchial tree at a positive pressure through a single tube, spasm of the cords may result in emphysema (see page 39), and in a rise of intrathoracic pressure which handicaps the circulation. If, however, a wide-bore tube is in place in the glottis when either insufflation or suction is applied, these dangers are circumvented, for there is free communication with the outside air, and neither positive nor negative pressure is brought to bear on the bronchial tree.

REFLEX EFFECTS OF INTUBATION

It has long been recognized[22] that intubation in light anaesthesia provokes reflex disturbances such as cough, breath-holding, and cyanosis. Reid and Brace[23] have investigated the behaviour of the circulatory system during intubation by electrocardiographic studies, and have reported several cases of arrhythmia which occurred either at the moment of intubation or of inflation of the cuff. They believe that such disturbances are more frequently seen in light anaesthesia, and that they are due to a reflex effect either upon the centres of the heart itself or upon the coronary arteries. In their opinion morphine tends to potentiate these effects, and atropine to inhibit them.

Inasmuch as intubation in light anaesthesia usually gives rise to disturbances of respiration frequently resulting in a temporary lack of oxygen, and since some of their cases occurred while using an agent which often, of itself, gives rise to such disturbances of the circulatory system, it is debatable whether intubation itself is responsible for them. The facts recorded by these authors, however, suggest a further reason for which intubation is better performed in deep than in light anaesthesia.

MECHANICAL COMPLICATIONS DURING MAINTENANCE

Several mechanical difficulties may occur during endotracheal anaesthesia, some of which have been referred to elsewhere.

It is never a safe assumption on the part of the anaesthetist that if intubation has been performed respiratory obstruction *cannot* occur and that he can therefore neglect to keep both the patient and the apparatus under constant supervision.

The Aspiration of Foreign Fluids.—If a patient is intubated without the use of an inflatable cuff or pharyngeal pack, any foreign matter in the pharynx may be aspirated into the respiratory tree during inspiration. This is less likely to occur if a slight positive pressure is in use, since the outflow of vapor between the tube and the glottis will tend to prevent it. Whenever an uncuffed tube is used as a laryngeal airway under a mask and without pharyngeal packing, aspiration is possible. The techniques permitting of such aspiration should therefore be avoided when there is any likelihood of vomiting during anaesthesia, or in any other case in which foreign fluids are likely to be present in the pharynx.

Kinking of the Tube.—All flexible tubes except those made of metal may become kinked in their course. The softer the tube the more likely is this complication. The more weight of apparatus is attached to the tube the greater becomes the probability that movements of the patient or the apparatus during maintenance may result in obstruction to respiration from this cause. Kinking of the tube can occur either in the pharynx or in the nasal fossa. Figure 37 is the lateral radiograph of the head and neck of a patient in whom nasotracheal intubation had been performed. It shows a kink almost completely obstructing the tube at the posterior choanae. Most kinks can be removed by manipulation of the tube. If this is unsuccessful, a stiffer tube must be used, or another route of intubation chosen. When the patient is in the supine position it is important to arrange the rubber tubing connecting the endotracheal tube to the source of vapor in such a way that the surgeons cannot lean upon it. This is a common cause of respiratory difficulty in operations upon the head, and one which often escapes the notice of the novice.

Biting of the Tube.—In oral intubation the tube must be protected from being bitten by the patient, otherwise complete respiratory obstruction will result. This is usually achieved by

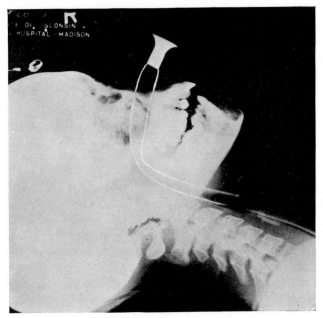

FIG. 37. RADIOGRAPH SHOWING KINKING OF A NASAL TUBE AT THE
POSTERIOR CHOANAE

The outline of the tube, though plainly visible in the original
X-ray, has had to be slightly retouched for purposes of repro-
duction.

placing a metal or gauze "bite-block" between the teeth when
oral intubation has been performed. The bite-block must, however, be watched, and replaced should it become displaced during the operation.

Separation of the Angle-Piece from the Tube.—It sometimes
happens, especially during long operations in which the head
is frequently moved, that the angle-piece slips out of the tube.
The tube is then loose, and can either be coughed out of the
trachea or be aspirated downwards into it. If the lubricating
vaseline finds its way in between the tube and the angle-piece
this accident is more likely to occur. The anaesthetist should
be aware of this possibility, which should occur to him whenever he observes any untoward leakage of vapor during endotracheal anaesthesia. Such an observation enables the trouble to

be rectified early. If the tube is completely disconnected and has slipped out of reach in the pharynx it must at once be re-covered—by laryngoscopy if necessary. A nasal tube which has become disconnected can sometimes be recovered in the nose by the gentle use of suitable forceps. Or the mouth may be opened wide and the tube withdrawn from the nasopharynx by hooking it forwards with the index finger. For these rea-sons it is wise, before intubation, to force the angle-piece into the tube so that it takes as firm a grip as possible.

DANGERS INHERENT IN THE USE OF COMPRESSED GASES

It is customary nowadays to use cylinders as the source of the gases used for anaesthesia. The cylinders are filled by com-pression of the gases, the usual pressure in a full cylinder being approximately two thousand pounds to the square inch. If by some accident such pressures should be brought to bear on the patient's respiratory tract, grave damage will ensue. One such case has been mentioned on page 40, and the dangers inherent in the use of positive pressure have been discussed on pages 112-115. Some workers have contended that the use of gases at high pressures is safe because in the event of an accident the anaesthetic apparatus will give way at a lower pressure than that at which mechanical damage to the patient will occur. This naturally depends upon the type of apparatus in use, but the argument is obviously unsound with respect to many mod-ern makes. Many workers use reducing valves on the cylinders. These reduce the high pressure in the cylinders to lower work-ing pressures. Certain types of reducing valve can be set to de-liver the gases at any pressure up to eighty pounds per square inch. The danger to the patient of an accidental release of gas at a high pressure is greater when endotracheal anaesthesia is in use. The anaesthetist must therefore be on his guard against the possibility. It is a wise precaution to use gases only at re-duced pressures; and if a reducing valve is not in use, to insist on turning on the cylinders himself, having first made certain that the fine adjustment valves are shut.

REFERENCES

1. HEWER, C. L. Brit. Jour. Anaes. 1923. I. 113.
2. TUFFIER, Th. and LOEWY, G.   La Presse Medicale, 1914. XXII. 497.
3. GUEDEL, A. E. and WATERS, R. M.   Curr. Res. Anaes. & Analg. 1928. VII. 238.
4. FLAGG, P. J.   The Art of Anaesthesia. 6th ed. Philadelphia, 1939. p. 148.
5. KING. F. G.   Curr. Res. Anaes. & Analg. 1940. XIX. 237.
6. GUEDEL, A. E. and TREWEEK, D. N.   Curr. Res. Anaes. & Analg. 1934. XIII. 263.
7. WATERS, R. M.   Proc. Roy. Soc. Med. (Anaes.) 1936. XXX. 11.
8. NOSWORTHY, M. D.   Proc. Roy. Soc. Med. (Surg.) 1940. XXXIV. 95.
9. TUFFIER, Th.   La Presse Medicale, 1906. XIV. 57.
10. BARACH, A. L., MARTIN, J., and ECKMAN, M.   Ann. Int. Med. 1938. XII. 754 (Vol. I).
11. MARCOTTE, R. J., PHILLIPS, F. J., ADAMS, W. E., and LIVINGSTONE, H. Jour. Thor. Surg. 1940. IX. 346.
12. ADAMS, W. E.   Jour. Thor. Surg. 1940. IX. 254.
13. HEIDRICK, A. F., ADAMS, W. E., and LIVINGSTONE, H.   Arch. Surg. 1940. XLI. 61.
14. GEORG, C.   Am. Jour. Surg. (Anaes. Supp.) 1917. XXXI. 77.
15. BRADSHAW, H. H.   Jour. Thor. Surg. 1939. VIII. 293.
16. MACKLIN, C. C.   C. M. A. J. 1937. XXXVI. 414.
17. ————Arch. Int. Med. 1939. LXIV. 913.
18. HALDANE, J. S. and PRIESTLY, J. G.   Respiration. 2d ed. Oxford, 1935. pp. 360-362.
19. EISENBREY, A. B.   Surg. Gyn. & Obs. 1912. XV. 715.
20. JANEWAY, H. H.   Ann. Surg. 1912. LVI. 328.
21. BARACH, A. L. in Barr's Modern Medical Therapy in General Practice. Baltimore, 1940. pp. 2478–2480.
22. QUINBY, W. C.   Surg. Gyn. & Obs. 1910. XI. 482.
23. REID, L. C. and BRACE, D. E.   Surg. Gyn. & Obs. 1940. LXX. 157.

VII. SEQUELAE OF ENDOTRACHEAL ANAESTHESIA AND THEIR INFLUENCE ON THE CHOICE OF ROUTE

INTUBATION may give rise to two varieties of complication, traumatic and infective. Either of these may be serious or slight. The literature contains a great deal of discussion of these possibilities, and the reports of certain isolated cases in which noteworthy sequelae have occurred. Much of the discussion has centered upon the choice of the route of intubation, and this has often obscured the main issue as to whether or not intubation itself increases the incidence of postoperative respiratory complications. Since the choice of route of intubation, where a choice exists, is largely conditioned by the results to be expected in the postoperative period, this question must be considered in relation to that of the sequelae of intubation. These issues will therefore be considered seriatim.

THE SEQUELAE OF INTUBATION
TRAUMATIC

The instrumentation of any orifice of the body is apt to engender minor traumatic sequelae; and the mouth, nose, pharynx, glottis, and trachea are no exception. Such occurrences do not, however, deter the medical profession from catheterizing the bladder or from dilating the cervix uteri, the rectum, or the oesophagus where an advantage to the patient may accrue. Nor should they discourage it from intubating the trachea in similar circumstances. The minor sequelae sometimes seen after intubation are tracheitis, laryngitis, pharyngitis, rhinitis, and mechanical damage to the teeth, nose, pharynx, or larynx.

It is evident, from conversations with individual workers, that several cases of grave trauma following intubation have not found their way into print. Anaesthetists are no more lacking in candor than their surgical colleagues; both know that occasional accidents inevitably occur in the performance of difficult operations, and that their publication may give rise to an unjustifiable prejudice against a useful proceeding. Intubation is no more to be condemned because the true cords have sustained permanent damage at the hands of an unskilled anaesthetist than is the dilatation of a malignant stricture of the oesophagus because, in inept hands, this operation has resulted in death from mediastinitis. Many authors have mentioned the incidence of minor traumatic sequelae of intubation in their hands; the figures are scarcely worth quoting, since they vary from two to eighty per cent. Almost all authors agree, however, that with intubation, as with all manual interventions on the human body, trauma can be avoided only by the acquisition of gentleness born of skill and experience.

"Acute oedema of the glottis" has been known to follow a traumatic intubation (see page 147). It is probably less uncommon in infants than in older patients, and is thought to be the result of infection superimposed upon mechanical trauma at intubation. The author has heard of a case of avulsion of a true cord by the forcible passage of a tube.

The literature contains records of nine cases of laryngeal granulomata following intubation. Griffith[1] has seen "five or six" cases in a series of fifteen hundred endotracheal anaesthetics, of which, apparently, the majority were by oral intubation. Clausen[2] reported a case in 1932, a granuloma being discovered five months after a difficult nasal intubation by direct vision. Gould[3] saw a similar case following an easy blind nasal intubation with a small tube for a lengthy operation. In this case the growth recurred after being removed once and required a second avulsion. Yet another case was reported by Cohen[4] in 1938. This occurred after a difficult blind nasal intubation. Another case, following oral intubation with a cuffed "anode" tube, has recently been reported by Smiley.[30] Where these growths were histologically examined they showed the characteristics of organized blood clots. Apparently, then, in certain rare cases, even a soft rubber tube can cause traumatic sequelae. The occurrence of emphysema after endotracheal anaesthesia has already been discussed on pages 39, and 112–115.

Lennon and Rovenstine[5] have reported a case in which death followed the rupture of an inflatable cuff inside a trachea the integrity of whose wall had already been impaired by pre-existing disease. The patient developed subcutaneous emphysema and died on the second day after operation. At autopsy there was found to be a break in the continuity of the mucosa of the right main bronchus, and this rupture occurred in an area of ulceration of the mucosa of long standing. This accident was therefore probably due to the coincidence of two rare phenomena: ulceration of the bronchus and rupture of the cuff.

Kaye[6] has suggested that the passage of a wide-bore tube is more likely to engender laryngitis than the use of a small-bore insufflation catheter. In a small series of cases he found that the incidence of minor complications after the passage of a wide-bore tube was 3.3 per cent, but only 2 per cent after the use of a small tube.

INFECTIVE

The "major" postoperative respiratory complications, such as pneumonia, acute bronchitis, empyema, and pulmonary abscess, are almost all infective in nature. They are the bugbear of surgeon and anaesthetist alike, and are responsible for a large number of deaths in the postoperative period. That many causes contribute to their incidence has been established in a great number of papers, the consideration of which is outside the scope of this work. They are especially common among patients of poor physical condition, and after certain types of operation. It is a well-established fact that in elderly patients a post-mortem finding of broncho- or hypostatic pneumonia is the rule rather than the exception. Such a finding is equally usual in patients who have undergone an operation, and in their case it is often labelled as an "ether pneumonia." The view is nevertheless gaining ground that the pulmonary lesion is only indirectly attributable to the effects of the anaesthetic, and that the condition of the patient and the type of operation performed directly influence its onset.

From the earliest days of endotracheal anaesthesia divergent views have been held as to the relation borne by the method to the incidence of these complications. Meltzer[7] practised endotracheal insufflation in dogs already suffering from a very fatal type of pneumonia, and found that none of the animals succumbed. The majority of workers, in the early days of insufflation, felt that the method gave rise to fewer respiratory sequelae than the alternatives then available. Elsberg[8] felt that insufflation was indicated in cases of chronic bronchitis, since it gave rise to no respiratory complications. In the intervening years many workers have expressed similar views. On the other hand, it has been suggested that intubation may contaminate the lower respiratory tract with organisms from the upper, and thus increase the incidence of respiratory sequelae. Tuffier and Loewy[9] suggested that insufflation tubes should be passed with their lumen filled with a stylet, so that the lumen of the tube should not become filled with secretions in its passage through the pharynx. Shipway[10] evidently considered infection from above possible, for he has pointed out that, if passed through the barrel of the laryngoscope, a tube is protected from contamination during its passage through the pharynx. Trotter[11] was the first surgeon to raise this objection to intubation. He was solely concerned with those cases in which an ulcerating malignant growth was present in the upper air passages, fearing that the lower respiratory tract might become infected by portions of such a growth which might be broken off and carried in during intubation. Shipway[12] replied to this objection by pointing out that no such case had as yet occurred.

The literature contains a wealth of opinion expressed by clinicians on this point, but scarcely any of these opinions are founded on the solid basis of recorded observations. Those who have ever had the opportunity to express an opinion on any technical point, and subsequently to verify it by reference to the recorded facts, know how entirely untrustworthy is the memory of any individual. No evidence, as distinct from opinion, has as yet been submitted touching the relation of intubation to the incidence of infective postoperative respiratory complications.

THE CHOICE OF ROUTE

The trachea may be intubated by way either of the mouth or of the nose. The popularity of the nasal route has been growing since 1930, and this has naturally revived the controversy over the relation of intubation to respiratory infection. Nasotracheal intubation has been adversely criticized by many authorities, and warmly defended by its exponents. There are three criteria by which the merits of either route may be assessed: (1) its practicability: the ease with which it may be achieved; (2) the facilities in working conditions which it provides; and (3) its sequelae. Of these the first two are chiefly of moment to the surgeon and the anaesthetist; the third is a matter of vital concern to the patient as well. Moreover, the sequelae of intubation are often the direct result of the ease with which it may be achieved. Thus the problem of the choice between the two routes is inseparable from a discussion of the sequelae of endotracheal anaesthesia.

In any operation upon the head or neck the surgeon's facility of access to the operative field is often the determining argument for the use of either route. When the site of the proposed operation is elsewhere in the body the anaesthetist is free to choose whichever route he considers the more desirable, and on this point opinions are sharply divided. Since there are advantages and disadvantages associated with the use of either route, neither should be used unthinkingly as a matter of "routine."

Magill has repeatedly stated that when confronted with the choice of route he prefers the nasal "because of the high percentage of cases in which the tube will enter the trachea without the aid of any instrument."[13] In another paper[14] he says, "the blind technique is so simple that it is always worth while exploring the possibilities of the nasal route when there is a free choice and when no contra-indications, such as sinus infection or gross nasal deformity, exist."

On the other hand the majority of anaesthetists still use the oral route wherever possible. Hewer,[15] Crafoord,[16] and Milne and Mackenzie[17] have all recently suggested that the nasal route should be avoided unless it must be used. Flagg[18] discusses only oral intubation in his book, and Griffith[1] clearly prefers the oral to the nasal route. Anaesthetists in Britain and Australia have exhibited a greater partiality for nasal intubation than have their colleagues in the United States and Canada.

Apparently the ease with which intubation can be performed by either route is almost entirely a matter of practice. In view of the fact that Magill used the laryngoscopic method of oral intubation in a very large number of cases before he evolved the blind nasal technique, we may well accept his view that, at worst, nasal intubation is no more difficult than oral, given equal experience. As one of a generation of anaesthetists who "grew up" professionally with both methods, the author feels that there is not much to choose between the two routes as regards the technical difficulties of intubation. Fortunately, as has been pointed out (pages 94–95), patients who are difficult to intubate by one route are often easy by the other. Never is the act of intubation so easy that it can be casually undertaken: to do so is to court serious trouble.

It is, however, by their sequelae that the relative merits of the two routes are to be judged, and, as we have seen, opinions differ on this point. The incidence of traumatic complications depends on the ease with which intubation can be accomplished. The advocates of the nasal route urge the following points as evidence that this route is less conducive to trauma: 1. In highly skilled hands, blind intubation is successful in ninety per cent of cases, and this makes further instrumentation superfluous. 2. A soft rubber tube is almost atraumatic. 3. Trauma to the teeth is entirely avoided.

Those who advocate the use of the oral route adduce the following arguments to show that oral intubation is less traumatic: 1. Every larynx should be visually examined before intubation in order to ascertain that it is normal.[19] 2. Laryngoscopy properly conducted is, or should be, atraumatic. 3. There is ample room for the passage of the tube without the danger of trauma to the structures. Anyone who has used both routes extensively will be aware that in each case only the third statement is true beyond question; and that these claims hold good only of the easy cases, since difficulties occur equally frequently with both routes. There is not much to choose between the inadvertent performance of adenoidectomy by nasal intubation and dental extraction by laryngoscopy!

It seems reasonable to suppose that if the transport of organisms from the upper to the lower respiratory tract plays any part in the incidence of respiratory complications after intubation, then nasal intubation should be more conducive to the establishment of such conditions than oral. Hornabrook[20] of Australia, in a spirited attack on superfluous intubation, stated his conviction that any intubation increased the risk of infective respiratory complications, and went so far as to quote a surgeon's description of nasal intubation as "a perfectly filthy method." In 1937 Dawkins[21] published a paper which is actually a plea for the more discriminating use both of endotracheal anaesthesia and of the nasal route. Unfortunately he confused the issue by comparing one series of cases in which intubation had not been performed with another series in which apparently all the patients had been intubated by the nasal route. He cited a case in which blind nasotracheal intubation was demonstrated by the anaesthetist at the close of a herniotomy in a healthy patient. The man died in forty-eight hours of bronchopneumonia, and at autopsy the same organism was found both in his nose and in the pulmonary lesions. Yet, dramatic as this sounds, it does not show that the organisms were present in the nose before operation. They may have been projected into it afterward during an attack of coughing. Dawkins' figures showed an incidence of major respiratory complications twice as high after nasotracheal intubation as when intubation was not performed; and the percentage of cases which ended fatally was also doubled. From this he argued that intubation itself was the cause of the higher morbidity and mortality, although he did not investigate the preoperative condition of the patients. There was no mention of orotracheal intubation, nor was it specifically stated that in all cases the nasal route was used. As there were no other figures available with which to compare those of Dawkins, the *British Journal of Anaesthesia* published, as an editorial symposium,[22] the views of a number of anaesthetists and one surgeon on intubation. None of these felt that naso-tracheal intubation gave rise to an increase in sequelae, provided that it was skilfully and judiciously used. They all agreed that any infectious process in the nasal passages was to be regarded as a contra-indication to nasal intubation, and that trauma at intubation was the most usual cause of postoperative complications. With the latter conclusion Dawkins[23] agreed, and quoted his statistics to the effect that when nasal intubation had succeeded at the first attempt the incidence of respiratory complications had been 3.9 per cent; but that this figure had risen to 10.7 per cent when two or more attempts had been required to perform intubation. Kelly,[24] who ever since 1912 has insisted on the use of insufflation methods in his cases, is a bitter opponent of the nasal route, believing that it is more likely to give rise to infections of the lower respiratory tract.

The results of 2,719 intubations have recently been statistically surveyed at the Wisconsin General Hospital.[25] The purpose of this investigation was to compare the incidence of sequelae after oral and nasal intubation; and about an equal number of patients had been intubated by either route. Table II shows the results of this investigation, and compares the incidence of complications following intubation by either route in normal patients and in subjects known to be suffering from respiratory disease before operation. The incidence of major complications is, if anything, lower after nasal than after oral intubation. These figures, therefore, do not substantiate the contention that serious sequelae are likely to follow nasal intubation. Every patient who died and exhibited signs of a major respiratory complication before death or at autopsy was classified as a "death following major complication." The incidence of these is lower after nasal than after oral intubation. On the other hand, these figures support the view of Magill[14] and others[26] that the nasal route is better avoided in patients suffering from pre-existing respiratory disorders. Indeed, in the entire series, the incidence of minor complications is uniformly higher after nasal than after oral intubation.

Many workers have assumed that the bulk of an inflatable cuff makes it unsuitable for use by the nasal route. The method has, however, been found practicable by Tovell,[27] Macintosh,[28] and Guedel.[29] Tovell designed, in 1936, a special cuffed tube intended for use by this route. It is difficult to be certain of the

TABLE II

A. PATIENTS WITHOUT PREOPERATIVE RESPIRATORY DISEASE
(1868 Cases)

	NASOTRACHEAL		OROTRACHEAL	
	No.	Per Cent	No.	Per Cent
Cases showing major complications after operation.........	34	3.7	50	5.2
Cases showing minor complications after operation.........	134	14.7	108	11.3
Cases showing no complications after operation	741	81.6	801	83.5
Total	909	100.0	959	100.0
Deaths following major complications	12	1.32	13	1.36

B. PATIENTS WITH PREOPERATIVE RESPIRATORY DISEASE
(851 Cases)

	NASOTRACHEAL		OROTRACHEAL	
	No.	Per Cent	No.	Per Cent
Cases showing major complications after operation.........	41	10.2	44	9.8
Cases showing minor complications after operation.........	102	25.3	54	12.2
Cases showing no complications after operation	260	64.5	350	78.0
Total	403	100.0	448	100.0
Deaths following major complications	15	3.7	22	4.9

position of the cuff in the trachea or glottis if blind intubation has been performed; and if laryngoscopy is resorted to the chief asset of the nasal route is lost.

To sum up the arguments for and against the use of either route, we may fairly decide:

1. To choose, unless there be good reason to the contrary, the route most convenient to the surgeon.

2. To choose whichever route seems to promise the easier and less traumatic intubation.

3. To avoid the nasal route in patients suffering from respiratory disease or nasal deformity.

4. To avoid the oral route in persons who have short thick necks and a full set of teeth; and in those with fragile teeth.

5. Never to yield to the temptation to overcome mechanical difficulties by the use of force instead of skill.

REFERENCES

1. GRIFFITH, H. R.   Curr. Res. Anaes. & Analg. 1932. XI. 206.
2. CLAUSEN, R. J.   Proc. Roy. Soc. Med. (Anaes.) 1932. XXV. 1507.
3. GOULD, R. B.   Brit. Med. Jour. 1935. II. 499.
4. COHEN, M.   Brit. Med. Jour. 1938. I. 283.
5. LENNON, B. B. and ROVENSTINE, E. A.   Curr. Res. Anaes. & Analg. 1939. XVIII. 217.
6. KAYE, G.   Brit. Jour. Anaes. 1936. XIII. 157.
7. MELTZER, S. J.   J. A. M. A. 1911. LVII. 521.
8. ELSBERG, C. A.   N. Y. State Jour. Med. 1912. XII. 524.
9. TUFFIER, Th. and LOEWY, G.   La Presse Medicale, 1914. XXII. 497.
10. SHIPWAY, F. E.   Proc. Roy. Soc. Med. (Anaes.) 1920. XIII. 1.
11. TROTTER, W.   Lancet, 1914. II. 1168.
12. SHIPWAY, F. E.   Lancet, 1914. II. 1274.
13. MAGILL, I. W.   Newcastle Med. Jour. 1934. XIV. 67.
14. ————Practitioner, 1933. CXXX. 430.
15. HEWER, C. L.   Recent Advances in Anaesthesia & Analgesia. 3d ed. Philadelphia, 1939. p. 117.
16. CRAFOORD, C.   On the Technique of Pneumonectomy in Man. Stockholm, 1938. p. 63.
17. MILNE, R. M. P. and MACKENZIE, J. R.   Brit. Med. Jour. 1939. II. 1136.
18. FLAGG, P. J.   The Art of Anaesthesia. 6th ed. 1939.
19. JACKSON, C.   Surg. Gyn. & Obs. 1913. XVII. 507.
20. HORNABROOK, F. W.   Curr. Res. Anaes. & Analg. 1931. X. 241.
21. DAWKINS, C. J. M.   Brit. Jour. Anaes. 1937. XIV. 45.
22. Editorial.   Brit. Jour. Anaes. 1937. XIV. 109.
23. DAWKINS, C. J. M.   Brit. Jour. Anaes. 1937. XIV. 182.
24. KELLY, R. E.   Brit. Med. Jour. 1940. I. 32.
25. GILLESPIE, N. A. and CONROY, W. A.   Anaesthesiology, 1941. II. 28.
26. LUNDY, J. S. and TUOHY, E. B.   Proc. Staff Meetings Mayo Clinic, 1937. XII. 225.
27. TOVELL, R. M.   Proc. Staff Meetings Mayo Clinic, 1936. XI. 565.
28. MACINTOSH, R. R.   Personal Communication. 1939.
29. GUEDEL, A. E.   Personal Communication. 1940.
30. SMILEY, W. A.   Ann. Otol. Rhinol. and Laryngol. 1940. XLIX. 556 and 572.

VIII. THE PRACTICAL APPLICATIONS OF ENDOTRACHEAL ANAESTHESIA

GENERAL CONSIDERATIONS

WE HAVE SAID that as a rule, and except for operations too short to justify the intubation, endotracheal anaesthesia is desirable in almost all interventions upon the head or neck. In these, and all other operations in the course of which the surgeons are wont to move the head upon the body during light endotracheal anaesthesia, the patient may resent the irritation of the movement of the tube in his trachea. This takes the form of retching or coughing, and results in movements which may seriously inconvenience the performance of a delicate operation, besides being unseemly. The use of the analgesic lubricants referred to on page 62 helps to overcome this difficulty. If they are not available these reactions can be minimized by directing down the lumen of the tube during inspiration the spray of a nebulizer containing one of the local analgesic solutions previously referred to (page 63).

In all operations on the head or neck the anaesthetist should find out where the surgeon and his assistants wish to stand, and should then arrange the anaesthetic apparatus so that it is as little in their way as possible. The angle-piece used to connect the tube may be made to point upward toward the forehead, downward toward the chest, or laterally, either from the nose or the mouth. The position which will allow the surgeon maximum freedom should be thought out beforehand, preferably after consultation with him.

It has already been pointed out (page 27) that asepsis in operations on the head has been greatly enhanced by the fact that intubation of the trachea in these patients makes further interference with the head by the anaesthetist superfluous during the operation. Nevertheless no assumption is more mistaken than that, when once a tube is in place, the anaesthetist can afford to ignore the respiratory movements. Tubes are subject to the accidents mentioned on pages 116–118; and the character of the respiration is the anaesthetist's chief criterion of the level of anaesthesia. Moreover, it is the anaesthetist's bounden duty closely and constantly to observe the behaviour of the patient's circulatory system. It is almost always possible so to arrange matters that a palpable pulse is within the reach of the anaesthetist. If the head is the site of operation either the radial pulse or that of the internal popliteal artery at the internal malleolus are available for the purpose. In any event the anaesthetist should be able to observe the blood pressure, the phonendoscope and sphygmomanometer for the purpose being provided with the necessary lengths of rubber tubing. Naturally, when a patient has been intubated, the anaesthetist is free to use his hands for other purposes than holding a mask on the face, and even to move about the room. The author has been enabled thereby, in a moment of emergency, to start a badly needed infusion of blood or fluid. This freedom, if wisely and conscientiously used, is a great asset; its abuse by the lazy or incompetent may lead to bad anaesthesia or even to the endangering of the patient's life.

We will now examine in detail the application of endotracheal anaesthesia to the different types of operations.

IN CEREBRAL OPERATIONS

Anaesthesia for these operations has always been a hotly debated subject, and one presenting grave technical difficulties. The patients are usually suffering from an increase in intra-cranial pressure; and when to this are added the inflictions of operation and anaesthesia, respiratory failure is liable to occur. Moreover, these patients often exhibit that form of vomiting which is associated with lesions of the brain. Therefore the complete control of the airway and the ability to exclude vomitus from the respiratory tract and to perform efficient artificial ventilation at a moment's notice provided by intubation are desirable. Cerebral operations demand strict asepsis, and thus it is advantageous if the anaesthetist can remain at a distance without losing his control of the airway. In many of the operations the patient is in a position which renders access to the face difficult and real control of the airway impossible without intubation. It is not surprising therefore that Elsberg[1] and Woolsey[2] applied the insufflation endotracheal technique to cerebral operations soon after its inception; and that Mennell[3, 4] used it extensively at the National Hospital in London. In those days the operations seldom exceeded three hours in duration, and ether was usually used. Gilbert Brown of Adelaide[5, 6] and Easson Brown of Toronto[7] have also reported favorably on the use of insufflation endotracheal ether anaesthesia; and for many years open ether anaesthesia, with an endotracheal inhalation tube in place under the mask, has been in use at the Mayo Clinic.[8] The growing influence of the Cushing school of cerebral surgeons has gradually led to a great increase in the duration of these operations, and electro-surgical methods are being used more and more. Both these trends have served to diminish the popularity of ether and to increase that of nitrous oxide as the agent of choice in these cases; and avertin, introduced in 1929, has been found to have qualities which make it a useful adjunct to nitrous oxide. Increasing experience, however, has merely served to confirm the view that, whatever agent is in use, the assurance of a free airway provided by intubation is of paramount importance. For some years endotracheal nitrous oxide–oxygen with minimal ether, with or without a preliminary basal narcosis with avertin, was regarded as the method of choice.[9, 10, 11, 12] The most recent tendency is to use nitrous oxide–oxygen endotracheally after basal narcosis with avertin.[13] With this technique, absolutely smooth anaesthesia can be secured without sub-oxygenation of the patient; and if the carbon dioxide absorption technique is resorted to for maintenance, both the smoothness and the economy of the method are greatly increased. To such an extent is this true that this technique appears to solve most of the difficulties of anaesthesia for cerebral operations.

Certain practical points in the management of the endotracheal method in cerebral cases deserve mention. Although either route of intubation may be used, the nasal is the more convenient for two reasons: deep anaesthesia is unnecessary for the operation, and blind intubation removes any necessity for it; and a tube in the nose is more easily and firmly secured in position than one in the mouth. Epistaxis on intubation is especially to be avoided in cerebral cases, for any blood in the tube is liable to clot during a long operation and obstruct the tube. This possibility must be watched for in any case in the prone position, for mucus can accumulate in the tube and cause a serious degree of obstruction. The breathing bag or tube amplifies sounds in the endotracheal tube. By placing the ear to the breathing bag or to the disconnected end of the accordion tube the rattle of any fluid in the endotracheal tube can be heard. Any fluid present should be removed by passing a small rubber catheter attached to a source of suction through the endotracheal tube. Lundy[14] recommends lubrication of the inside of the endotracheal tube to facilitate this. If the tube should become obstructed it must naturally be removed and replaced by a fresh one. While this sounds a formidable undertaking in the course of a cerebellar exploration, it has been found[12] that if a fresh tube is passed at once through the same nostril it frequently re-enters an open glottis with ease.

The separation of the angle-piece from the tube as described on page 117 is frequently seen during these long cases in the course of which much movement of the head occurs. In cerebral cases more than any others the tube is liable to be pulled out during the inevitable movement of the patient as he is placed in position on the operating table. The anaesthetist should never loose his hold on the tube while the patient is being moved, and it is wise entirely to disconnect the tube from the source of vapor at this time. Occasionally a surgeon requests that the induction be carried out in the sitting position. Either blind intubation or laryngoscopy at first seems difficult in this position because there is a tendency to extend the head without also moving it forward on the neck. With a little practice this art is soon mastered.

It has been suggested[11] that the presence of a tube in the nose for as long as twelve or fifteen hours might give rise to an oedema of the Eustachian cushions, and so lead to an acute suppurative otitis media. As yet no such cases have been reported in the literature, although they have been observed.[15] They occurred, however, during an epidemic of streptococcal otitis media, and were probably not related to the intubation.

IN OTO-RHINO-LARYNGOLOGICAL OPERATIONS

In no field of surgery is true understanding and cooperation between surgeon and anaesthetist more valuable than here: it can make or mar the entire operation. Stupidity or lack of imagination and understanding on the part of the anaesthetist can easily mean death or grave complications to the patient. Surgeons experienced in the use of endotracheal anaesthesia in operations of this kind readily acknowledge their indebtedness to it.[16]

For the sake of convenience we will consider under this heading the plastic operations on the face and the superficial operations on the neck; and we will include the major dental operations under the heading of "operations in the mouth."

Operations upon the ear are conveniently performed with endotracheal anaesthesia. The beginner should remember, however, that if the surgeon usually takes fifteen minutes to perform cortical mastoidectomy, it is scarcely worth while to expend forty minutes in performing intubation. Acute mastoiditis is the condition par excellence in which the argument against nasal intubation on the grounds of a possible transport of infection might be justified; for these cases are usually caused by a virulent organism, and the pus tends to drain down the Eustachian tube into the nasal cavity. Often it is found in the pharynx as well. It seems reasonable, therefore, to avoid a nasal intubation in a patient with acute mastoiditis. When orotracheal intubation is used the tube can be protected from contamination by the barrel of the laryngoscope until it actually enters the glottis. In radical mastoidectomy and in the "Duel-Ballance" operation for the radical cure of facial paralysis,[17, 18] endotracheal anaesthesia is of great service, for it enables the anaesthetist to be out of the surgeons' way and yet to maintain smooth light anaesthesia and a complete control of the airway during a lengthy operation. Since only very light anaesthesia is required, nasal intubation by the blind technique seems ideal and provides excellent results. If infectious processes are still at work in the middle ear, the nostril on the diseased side should be avoided. If local analgesia of the trachea is practised, anaesthesia can usually be satisfactorily maintained with nitrous oxide. For reasons of mechanical convenience, as pointed out on page 110, the "semiclosed" method of maintenance is ideal in these superficial operations on the head and neck.

Endotracheal anaesthesia has revolutionized the operating conditions within the nasal cavity. Without it, anaesthesia was induced to as deep a plane as possible. The surgeon then packed the posterior nares with gauze or a sponge; and the anaesthetist inserted a pharyngeal airway and strove to maintain anaesthesia through it by the insufflation of vapor. Usually this did not succeed, even when the sheet was drawn up over the end of the airway and chloroform was poured upon it. The surgeon attempted to perform the operation with the patient moving about (he frequently had to be held down) and with frothy blood pouring out of the nostrils at each expiration, since the nasal pack was seldom free of leaks. Blood and pus therefore frequently found their way into the trachea. The anaesthesia was so light that the patient usually coughed them up, but the violent coughing did nothing to improve the operating conditions. Only those who have endured this state of affairs, in which blood poured from the nose to the table, from the table to the anaesthetist's apron, and from there to the floor, will fully appreciate the advantages conferred by endotracheal anaesthesia. Induction is performed, followed by orotracheal intubation either with a cuffed tube or a pharyngeal pack. The operation then proceeds unhurried and with adequate haemostasis, respiration having been entirely confined to the tube. Nasotracheal intubation is obviously contra-indicated; and "combined" operations such as the "Caldwell-Luc" type of drainage of the maxillary antrum, can be performed without hindrance from an oral tube. If an inflatable cuff is used it is well to remember that it does not always prevent blood from running down the oesophagus, and that if blood enters the stomach it is liable to cause postoperative vomiting. A gauze pack is the remedy.

In the various operations performed in the cavity of the pharynx, endotracheal anaesthesia is of great value; but its application calls for common sense and an intimate knowledge of the surgical requirements. The commonest operation in the pharynx is tonsillectomy, and the following case illustrates the need for both these attributes:

A throat surgeon, when asked why he seemed bad-tempered at lunch time, furnished the following explanation. He was to perform tonsillectomy and adenoidectomy upon the child of very wealthy parents. The latter had insisted upon the services of a distinguished anaesthetist who was, however, unacquainted with the surgeon or his habits. The anaesthetist arrived an hour before the operation was to start and administered a basal narcosis with avertin. He then performed induction of anaesthesia with nitrous oxide and ether, after which he expended a further thirty minutes in unsuccessful attempts at blind nasal intubation. Finally intubation was accomplished by direct vision. The surgeon then removed the tonsils in about one minute with a "Sluder" guillotine, and had to request the removal of the endotracheal tube in order to remove the adenoids. This was accomplished in a further half minute. This ludicrous combination of techniques could have been avoided had the anaesthetist paused to inquire of the surgeon what type of operation he intended to perform.

It is rarely worth intubating a child in whom the guillotine operation is to be performed, unless the surgical technique includes very deliberate haemostasis, so that the operation lasts ten minutes or more. Where dissection of the tonsils is performed in children the advisability of intubation is largely a matter of the known ability of the surgeon to maintain an unobstructed airway during the operation. If the airway is kept free perfectly satisfactory anaesthesia can be secured by an induction to the third plane of the third stage, and maintenance with ether by endopharyngeal insufflation. Many tonsillectomies are performed by young and inexperienced surgeons who are too absorbed in their own local difficulties to spare the necessary attention to keeping the airway clear. In such cases intubation is of value. Nasotracheal intubation is usually resorted to, but has certain disadvantages. In the author's experience, the patient with hypertrophied tonsils usually also has distortion of the nasal passages which makes nasal intubation difficult. This is true both in children and in adults. In children adenoidectomy is usually performed as well as tonsillectomy; and generally a nasal tube must be removed before this second part of the operation, since only a few surgeons can perform adenoidectomy without serious inconvenience from its presence. Oral intubation is free from this disadvantage, but an oral tube, even if pulled into the opposite angle of the mouth, can inconvenience the surgeon during tonsillectomy and is liable to be kinked or displaced by his movements.

Clement and McCarthy[19, 20] have found endotracheal methods valuable in tonsillectomy performed by dissection in the sitting position. In the adult, dissection of the tonsils and meticulous haemostasis are the rule and adenoidectomy is seldom performed. Smooth anaesthesia is almost impossible to maintain by pharyngeal insufflation. Nasotracheal intubation furnishes excellent results in these patients as Challis[21] has pointed out. He was concerned, however, with the surgical technique usual in England, where the head is placed in the "Rose" position, with the surgeon seated at the head of the table, and the patient's mouth opened wide by means of the "Boyle-Davis Gag."[22] The tube lies almost in the middle line of the pharynx and does not hinder the surgeon. Pharyngeal packing cannot be used in these cases, and therefore either a cuffed tube is passed or else the surgeon, before beginning to operate, places a small gauze pack in the hypopharynx so as to occlude the glottic opening around the tube. The anaesthetist should be careful that no positive pressure is used during maintenance, inasmuch as this greatly increases the venous oozing at the site of operation (see page 114).

In haemorrhage from the pharyngeal walls from any cause intubation is of value. In civil practice the commonest cause of this condition is inadequate haemostasis during tonsillectomy. Patients suffering from this condition are difficult to intubate because they have usually received large doses of morphine beforehand, so that the respiration is greatly depressed, and because the pharynx is obstructed by blood. This may also have found its way into the trachea. Intubation will permit the anaesthetist to remove the blood from the trachea by suction (see page 152) to prevent the entry of further blood, and to maintain smooth anaesthesia while the surgeon secures haemostasis. The author has been called upon to deal with a similar situation resulting from haemorrhage from the lingual artery after the insertion of radium into a carcinoma of the tongue.

Similar problems attend the choice of anaesthesia for operations upon malignant growths of the pharynx. Obviously, if the use of the diathermy is contemplated, non-inflammable agents must be used. The chief difficulty as regards intubation is the possibility of breaking off a fragment of the growth with the tube or laryngoscope and depositing it in the lower respiratory tract, where it may cause either infection or metastasis (see page 123). This possibility is not so much a reason for avoiding intubation as for performing it under direct vision with full relaxation, so that trauma does not occur.

The drainage of retropharyngeal abscesses is regarded by many as so dangerous that no anaesthetic should be employed. Many deaths have occurred as the result of this operation. The structures of the neck are inflamed and oedematous, and there is usually sufficient swelling to cause an obstruction to respiration. In these circumstances the evacuated pus increases this obstruction and may easily be inhaled. It would seem, therefore, that intubation is a valuable safeguard against both these accidents. It is likely to be difficult because of the local inflammation. Individual cases differ so much that academic discussion is futile, for each case must be judged at the time in the light of its own peculiar circumstances. If intubation is decided upon, the anaesthetist must be careful not to rupture the abscess during intubation. As a precaution against this accident the table should be placed in the "Trendelenburg" position before intubation. In every case of retropharyngeal abscess, however, the possibility of intubation should be carefully considered before being dismissed.

The operation of oesophagoscopy is greatly facilitated by the exhibition of endotracheal anaesthesia. The line taken by a nasal tube from the posterior choanae to the glottis crosses the line of passage of the oesophagoscope from the mouth to the cricoid sphincter forwards from behind. Therefore its presence may complicate the insertion of his instrument by the surgeon if he is unused to it. This mechanical difficulty is illustrated in Figure 38, which shows the lateral radiograph of the pharynx of a patient in whom an oesophagoscope is being inserted, a nasal tube being in place. The tip of the oesophagoscope is just beyond the cricoid sphincter, and the course of the nasal endotracheal tube has been emphasized by passing an opaque ureteric catheter through it. In the more delicate proceedings, such as the dilatation and intubation of malignant strictures of the oesophagus, or the implantation of radon seeds into them, as described by Souttar,[23, 24] nasotracheal anaesthesia is valuable, and

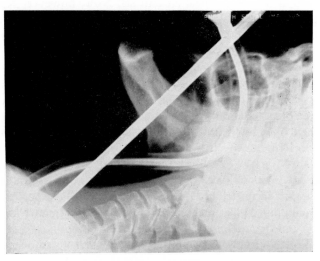

FIGURE 38.—RADIOGRAPH SHOWING THE PASSAGE OF AN OESOPHAGO-
SCOPE TO THE LEFT OF A NASAL TUBE IN PLACE

has been consistently used in his cases for many years. Other workers prefer orotracheal intubation. This enables the surgeon to pass his instrument more easily; but the tube must be carefully watched lest it become kinked or displaced by the surgeon's movements.

Oesophagoscopy undertaken for the recovery of a foreign body, however, presents different problems, especially if the foreign body is sharp and has lodged above the level of the fifth thoracic vertebra. In these cases unskilled attempts at blind nasotracheal intubation are dangerous and can provoke fatal consequences. For if the tube is pushed down into the oesophagus by mistake it may press upon the foreign body and cause it to puncture the wall of the oesophagus. A fatal mediastinitis may result from such a puncture. In these cases, then, the anaesthetist is wise to inquire as to the nature and location of the foreign body; and he should so plan his intubation that the tube is never allowed to enter the oesophagus.

Until recently there was unanimous agreement with Magill's statement[25] that operations upon the larynx itself are a contra-indication to endotracheal anaesthesia. Now, however, Nesbit and Waters[26] have found that intubation can be of service to the laryngologist in the removal of pedunculated papillomata of the larynx. Unless very deep anaesthesia with complete paralysis of the cords is attained, it can be difficult for the surgeon to reach the bases of the growths with the punch forceps for their removal. If a small endotracheal tube is passed and some degree of insufflation pressure is applied to the gases, the cords are held open by the tube and the return flow of the gases blows the growths out towards the surgeon, making them more accessible.

In other operations involving the larynx normal intubation is out of the question. Laryngectomy is usually preceded by tracheotomy. When this has been done an endotracheal anaesthetic can be administered through the tracheotomy opening. A tube of appropriate bore is cut short so that it can be passed into the tracheotomy wound without entering a bronchus. Either it should be fitted with an inflatable cuff or the surgeon should pack gauze between the tube and the tracheal walls, so that blood cannot be aspirated into the bronchi. This is the easiest form of endotracheal anaesthesia, for it obviates the difficulties of intubation.

Bronchoscopy does not admit of laryngeal intubation by the anaesthetist. Most bronchoscopes, however, are provided with a side-tube for the administration of gases, and by this artifice insufflation endotracheal anaesthesia can be maintained, the bronchoscope itself guaranteeing the patency of the return airway. The minute bulbs with which the Jackson instruments are illuminated can under certain conditions develop sufficient heat to ignite inflammable vapors. The latter are therefore better avoided for purposes of this operation.

In 1927 Magill[27] made a plea for the increased use of endotracheal anaesthesia in dental operations, and this has borne fruit with the passage of the years. Dental operations likely to last for less than fifteen minutes can be satisfactorily performed with nasal inhalation methods, and intubation is superfluous. Where maintenance for more than fifteen minutes is required the patient is best intubated by the nasal route, as Christiansen and McCarthy have pointed out.[28] The anaesthesia must be sufficiently deep to permit of opening the mouth at the beginning of the operation; and the usual precautions against the aspiration of blood should be taken. This technique is equally useful in plastic operations upon the mouth or lips, and in interventions inside the mouth, such as glossectomy or the removal of a ranula.

In all operations upon the neck with the exception of thyroidectomy (see page 143) endotracheal anaesthesia is of value. In certain cases it may enable the anaesthetist to assist the surgeon by demonstrating, from inside the pharynx, the position of the oesophagus, of the foramen caecum, or of an oesophageal diverticulum.

IN OPHTHALMIC OPERATIONS

Such a large proportion of the operations of ophthalmology are performed with local analgesia that ophthalmologists and anaesthetists seldom meet. Thus, unfortunately, there tends to be less mutual understanding of each other's problems, and therefore less co-operation between surgeon and anaesthetist, in this than in any other branch of surgery.

In all operations in which either of the chambers of the eye is opened it is essential that nothing shall occur which may raise the intra-ocular tension. Otherwise the aqueous or vitreous contents may be forced out, and the eye be lost. Vomiting, straining, coughing, and retching all cause an increase in the intra-ocular tension. Since the absence of all these before, during, and after endotracheal anaesthesia is improbable, it follows that the method should not be used in such cases.

In the other ophthalmic operations, however, this objection does not obtain, and endotracheal anaesthesia is as valuable as in other operations upon the head. The use of this technique abolishes most of the distaste which ophthalmologists of the older school feel for inhalation anaesthesia. This was chiefly inspired by the inconvenience of being hampered at every turn during the operation by the anaesthetist and his equipment. Anaesthesia should be maintained in the second plane of the third stage because the oscillatory movements of the eye which are characteristic of the first plane can seriously incommode the surgeon in his work.

It is to be hoped that in the future anaesthetists may be of more assistance to ophthalmic surgeons, for probably both the comfort and safety of their patients would benefit thereby. The present tendency to use local analgesia with or without heroic doses of non-volatile anaesthetic agents in all operations about the eye seems somewhat exaggerated. In cases of strabismus, dacryocystitis, and ectropion and for the operations of enucleation, evisceration, and exenteration of the orbit there is a large and fruitful field for the application of endotracheal anaesthesia. Either route of intubation may be used, the oral being probably the more convenient inasmuch as the tube will then be further removed from the field of operation.

IN THYROIDECTOMY

Thyroid operations fall into three categories from the standpoint of the anaesthetist: those performed primarily for the relief of respiratory obstruction, those intended for the treatment of thyrotoxicosis, and those undertaken chiefly for cosmetic reasons.

As early as 1902 Floren,[29] a pupil of Kühn, pointed out the value of intubation in thyroid operations complicated by respiratory obstruction. It would be tedious to enumerate all those who, in the intervening years, have agreed with him. Suffice it to say that all workers are agreed that where obstruction to respiration exists, intubation should be resorted to; and that during any thyroidectomy the anaesthetist should be prepared to intubate at once should obstruction supervene. Gross distortion and oedema of the structures are often present in such cases and may prove formidable obstacles to intubation.

It seems almost superfluous to point out that the tube must be placed deeply enough to relieve any obstruction with certainty, and that it must be of a material sufficiently resistant to withstand the pressure upon it. The following case illustrates the need for care in these respects:

A female patient in the fifth decade of life was to undergo removal of a cystic adenoma of the thyroid. A nitrous oxide–oxygen–ether induction was smoothly performed, and a smooth and very skilful blind nasal intubation followed. A No. 6 Magill tube of about the normal length was used. The patient, however, did not breathe again, and began to show cyanosis. The surgeon came into the room, saw the patient's color, and immediately made an incision in the neck and punctured the cyst-adenoma, allowing the fluid to escape. In the meantime the anaesthetist was making unavailing efforts to inflate the lungs with oxygen through the tube. The cyanosis increased progressively and the patient died. To the bystander it seemed evident that the rubber tube had become impacted in and compressed by the portion of the trachea constricted by the pressure of the gland.

The wisdom or otherwise of intubating the trachea in cases of thyrotoxicosis is a hotly debated subject. The patients are often poor anaesthetic risks: they tolerate deep anaesthesia badly and frequently exhibit respiratory complications in the postoperative period. Many exhibit before operation some degree of irritative tracheitis from the pressure of the gland. For these reasons it seems undesirable to subject them to the further irritation of surgical interference with the trachea while a tube is in place inside that structure. On the other hand, there are certain mechanical advantages to be derived from intubation. Patients suffering from thyrotoxicosis exhibit certain characteristic phenomena during operation: there is usually a sharp rise in the systolic pressure and pulse rate, and often in the pulse pressure as well, during surgical stimulus. This reaches a peak during traction on the gland, and usually subsides either when the vessels are ligated or when the lobe is actually removed. Then, if the other lobe is pulled upon, similar phenomena make their appearance, to subside again during the process of suturing. The intensity of these changes appears to vary directly as the metabolic rate of the patient before operation; and during operation his consumption of oxygen appears to rise and fall with the pulse rate and blood pressure. The intensity of these phenomena depends to some extent upon the gentleness exhibited by the surgeon; for if he exerts great traction upon the gland in the light anaesthesia which is customary for this operation, reflex spasm of the glottis occurs. The lack of oxygen and excess of carbon dioxide to which this gives rise enhance the variations in pulse rate and blood pressure, and these may well cause the patient more harm than would a skilful intubation. Naturally it is difficult to maintain either smooth anaesthesia or adequate oxygenation of a patient under these conditions. Endotracheal anaesthesia can minimize these variations and ensure smoothness at the price of a slightly greater depth of anaesthesia. For this reason the technique has been used by many surgeons and anaesthetists ever since the early days of insufflation. Kelly[30] considers it the ideal method, and Joll[31] has used it routinely in a large number of cases. In 1927 Dunhill[32] stated his opinion that the use of endotracheal anaesthesia did not increase the incidence of respiratory complications after thyroidectomy. At that time Featherstone disagreed with this view. In more recent years Hewer and Keynes[33] have published figures which suggest that fatal respiratory complications are indeed somewhat higher in cases of thyroidectomy after intubation; and Lewis[34] felt that endotracheal anaesthesia was not justifiable in thyroidectomy performed for thyrotoxicosis. Waters[35] has suggested another reason for which intubation is better avoided. He believes that, provided the anaesthetist maintains a sufficiently light plane of anaesthesia, he can tell by the onset and character of the irritability of the cords that the surgeon is traumatizing the vicinity of the recurrent laryngeal nerve and can issue a warning in time to prevent him from dividing it. This naturally is impossible if the patient has been intubated. On the other hand Lahey[36] prefers that his patients be intubated, and relies on the exposure and identification of the nerve to prevent damage to it. This is primarily a matter for the surgeon, and therefore the decision whether to intubate a patient before thyroidectomy calls for a full comprehension, by both surgeon and anaesthetist, of all the factors involved in it.

The problem of whether thyrotoxic patients should be intubated turns on these points. If the surgeon is gentle in his manipulations, it should be possible to produce smooth anaesthesia without subjecting an already irritable trachea to the further insult of intubation. If the surgeon is rough, then the anaesthetist must decide which is more damaging to the patient: the stormy anaesthesia, with bouts of coughing, spasm, and cyanosis, or the intubation which will ensure smoothness at the price of somewhat deeper anaesthesia and the possibility of increased irritation of the trachea.

Patients suffering from enlargements of the thyroid gland which are neither toxic nor obstructive are easy to anaesthetize without intubation; but in them the most cogent reasons against intubation do not arise.

Peterson and Rovenstine[37] have reported a case in which intubation was performed for the relief of obstruction caused by a collapse of the trachea in the course of thyroidectomy. It was found that a Magill tube would not pass the site of the obstruction, and intubation was therefore performed with a semi-rigid tube. This was allowed to remain in place for six hours after the end of the operation and was removed when the patient began to resent its presence. Forty minutes after extubation respiratory obstruction again supervened and the tube was re-inserted. The patient, however, remained unconscious and died eight hours later. These facts suggest that the equipment for intubation should be ready for immediate use during any thyroidectomy; and that there are occasions on which the use of a semi-rigid tube is necessary.

IN OPERATIONS UPON INFANTS AND CHILDREN

During the discussion of a paper on anaesthesia in children in 1925, Magill and Clausen[38] both expressed their regret that the advantages of endotracheal anaesthesia were so seldom exploited in operations upon children. Probably the chief reason is that in comparatively few of these is the method required. Besides, intubation is technically more exacting in the child than the adult, and the difficulty varies inversely as the size of the child.

The difficulties of intubation originate partly from anatomical causes and partly from the behaviour of infants towards anaesthetics. The glottis is naturally small, and its protective reflex is extremely irritable, a condition appropriate to anyone who lives on liquids only. The epiglottis is proportionately longer than in the adult and appears to lie very close to the glottic opening. This is probably because the larynx occupies a higher position in the infant.[39] The ideal conditions for laryngoscopy (see page 67) cannot always be safely attained in infants because, whereas mandibular relaxation occurs early in anaesthesia, the glottic reflex may still be present when the circulatory or respiratory systems begin to show signs of intolerance of the depth of anaesthesia.[40] When laryngoscopy must be undertaken in the presence of an active glottic reflex, it is usually found that the glottis moves anteriorly with each breath and disappears from the field of vision. When the tube is passed, as Kaye[41] has pointed out, the infant is apt "to suffer from an intense respiratory spasm as soon as intubation has been performed. This spasm causes much anoxaemia and even when oxygen has been given is apt to leave the circulation depressed." Gentleness of manipulation, which is the only way to avoid the sequelae of intubation, is doubly important in dealing with the very delicate structures of an infant, as the following case shows:

A skilful and distinguished anaesthetist kindly undertook to replace the usual anaesthetist to a children's hospital. He had had a wide experience of intubation in adults, but little or none in infants. He was confronted with a baby six weeks old who was to have a hare-lip repaired. Induction and intubation occupied seventy-five minutes, after which the operation was performed in a further seventy-five minutes. Twelve hours later the child developed signs of obstructed respiration. A laryngologist was requested to see the case, performed laryngoscopy, and found an acute oedema of the glottis. As the obstruction was almost complete, he performed tracheotomy. The child recovered, the tracheotomy opening was subsequently closed, and the child survived to undergo the closure of the cleft palate a year later.

This possibility is always present when instrumentation of the glottis is performed in the infant, even by the most skilful workers. When the more traumatic proceeding of bronchoscopy is undertaken, some surgeons insist that a tracheotomy set be kept next to the child's bed for the next two days.[42] The oedema is commonly supposed to be due to a streptococcal infection brought about by the entrance of this organism into some small abrasion of the mucosa at the time of operation. For this reason it is wise to insist that cultures taken from the patient's throat be negative for streptococci and Klebs-Loeffler bacilli before these operations are performed.

The maintenance of anaesthesia presents certain mechanical difficulties even after intubation has been performed. An infant is easily exhausted by the effort of overcoming any resistance to respiration, and its tidal respiration is so small that excesses of carbon dioxide are easily built up in any closed system.

Ayre [43, 44] has made a valuable contribution by pointing out these possibilities and by suggesting a form of "injection inhalation" endotracheal system whereby they can be avoided. This consists of a T-tube, of which one limb is connected to the endotracheal tube, the middle limb to the source of vapor, and the other left open to the air. The child thus breathes back and forth into the open limb, while ether vapor is admitted to the system from the side-tube. If a piece of rubber is attached to the open limb, it should be kept sufficiently short to avoid an accumulation of carbon dioxide. Thus far these mechanical difficulties have prevented the application of the carbon dioxide absorption technique to anaesthesia in infants.

Nasotracheal intubation is fortunately rarely necessary in infants, for it is more difficult to perform than in adults. There is usually a hyperplasia of the "adenoid tissue," and gross deflection of the tube from its proper course is the rule rather than the exception. Any restriction of the lumen of their already small airway is to be avoided in these subjects, and there is little space available in the nose of an infant. Epistaxis is easily provoked and is often profuse. Finally, blind intubation is more difficult and less often successful in infants than in adults.[40] For these reasons it is wise to avoid the nasal in favor of the oral route whenever possible in the infant.

In the infant of less than one year certain plastic operations call for endotracheal methods. The repair of a hare-lip is the commonest of these, but congenital deformities or disfigurations of the face are sometimes encountered. The patients suffering from a hare-lip are often in a state of gross malnutrition, and may be of very small size. The author's smallest case weighed six pounds four ounces. Orotracheal intubation is usually used because the presence of a tube in the nostril causes some degree of distortion of the soft parts and therefore prejudices the accuracy of the suture line. Operations upon the palate are often undertaken in very young children, and some workers prefer nasotracheal anaesthesia for this operation.[45] Obviously, not only the route of intubation but the necessity for it depends mainly on the details of the surgical technique. The shorter and more superficial the operation, and the more careful the surgeon to maintain unobstructed respiration, the less need is there for intubation.

Operations for the open correction of torticollis are usually performed in children. Intubation often presents difficulties by either route because of the distortion of the structures inherent in the condition. Any lack of oxygen or excess of carbon dioxide during induction will promote muscular spasm and aggravate this distortion. The value of intubation in these cases, in which it is not essential, is debatable. It facilitates maintenance, operation, and the application of a plaster cast (Figure 39); but the perfect airway resulting from intubation may mislead the anaesthetist. Sometimes when the tube is removed it is found that the position of the head in the plaster gravely obstructs respiration. If intubation is not resorted to this fact will be noticed at the time (see page 102). The use of endotracheal anaesthesia in tonsil-

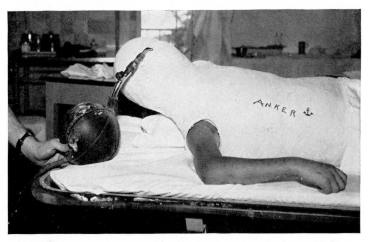

FIGURE 39.—THE CLOSE OF AN OPERATION FOR TORTICOLLIS WITH NASOTRACHEAL
ANAESTHESIA

This is the ideal method of anaesthesia for these operations. The area of the mouth and nose is covered with cotton wool and kept free from plaster of Paris, and a bite-block is in place in the mouth. Should the patient vomit during the application of the plaster the tube guarantees freedom of respiration, and the pharynx can be drained by suction.

lectomy in children has already been mentioned (page 136). Finally, it is usually required in cerebral operations. In children the management of these does not differ greatly from those in adults, discussed on pages 131–134.

Both the size of the glottis and the length of the trachea vary widely in infants and children,[30] and no rules can be laid down in advance. Whenever a child is to be intubated, a range of tubes of all reasonable sizes should be laid out ready for use. The largest possible size should then be used for the first attempt at intubation. If this proves too large, the next smaller size is tried. No force should ever be used in attempting to insert the tube. In the child partial occlusion of the respiratory passages is of more vital importance than in the adult, and the danger of intubating the right main bronchus by mistake is greater. The tube should be roughly measured beforehand by laying it alongside the child's neck and making sure that its length, measured from the incisor teeth in orotracheal, and from the nares in nasotracheal intubation, does not permit its end to reach the level of the second costal cartilage. The child's respirations should be closely watched after intubation. If any anomalies are observed their cause should be determined and removed before the operation is begun.

IN THORACIC OPERATIONS

Operations upon the thorax involve demands upon the anaesthetist not encountered in other special branches of surgery. The act of intubation itself is more difficult in these than in most cases. In many of them the effective area of the lungs available for the exchange of gases has been reduced by the processes of disease, and in many more the presence of secretion both impedes the freedom of airway and renders the respiratory passages irritable. The result is that the process of induction to a point at which intubation becomes easy is slow and difficult. Curiously enough almost all thoracic operations are still performed with the patient in the lateral position with the diseased lung uppermost. This throws upon the patient the strain of respiration under circumstances in which much of the weight of the body must be lifted with each inspiration. The institution of controlled respiration enables the anaesthetist to spare the patient much of this exertion by assuming it for him. The techniques of intubation to be discussed are more exacting than the simple intubation of the trachea, and should not be undertaken until the individual has mastered the more elementary proceeding. Thoracic surgery itself is still in its infancy, and the major operations, such as lobectomy and pneumonectomy, are as yet rarely performed. It follows that the methods of anaesthesia described are also tentative and experimental, for thus far few individuals have experienced more than a few cases at first hand. This is particularly true of the technique described as "endobronchial" intubation, upon which the opinions of the most experienced workers with endotracheal intubation differ sharply. We will consider in turn the various special difficulties which beset the anaesthetist in operations upon the thorax, and the measures by which they may be overcome. Then we will discuss the application of these principles to special operations.

THE CONTROL OF FOREIGN FLUIDS OR SUBSTANCES
IN THE RESPIRATORY PASSAGES

Many candidates for thoracic operations suffer from excessive secretions. These can be of sufficient volume to cause the death of the patient by drowning unless they can be removed during operation. In certain instances this drowning can happen with dramatic suddenness, as is illustrated by the following case:

A man of fifty-five was to undergo the drainage of an abscess in the lower lobe of the right lung. The young anaesthetist realized the possible dangers, but did not know how to prevent them. He administered a semiclosed nitrous oxide–chloroform anaesthesia because the diathermy was to be used, and performed blind intubation of the trachea. The surgeon then removed one rib over the site of the abscess, and, inserting a finger, he probed violently into the lung tissue in search of the abscess. Quite suddenly the patient developed gross cyanosis, his pupils dilated widely, his respirations ceased, and pus began to drip from the expiratory valve of the apparatus on the floor. The anaesthetist hastily turned the table into the Trendelenburg position, withdrew the endotracheal tube, and, snatching up a bronchoscope lying on an adjacent table, inserted it into the trachea and aspirated a large quantity of foul pus. It was too late, however. The patient was dead: drowned by the large volume of pus which was released when the surgeon's manipulations ruptured the abscess.

In operations upon the lung itself fragments of tissues of various kinds may be aspirated from the diseased lung into the trachea or the opposite lung. The removal of fluids is encompassed by the use of suction through a small catheter, which may be passed either alongside or through the endotracheal tube. Even fragments of tissue can sometimes be dislodged by this means. At no time, however, must suction drainage of the trachea or bronchi be resorted to unless an endotracheal tube or bronchoscope is in position. Otherwise a partial or massive collapse of the lungs may result (pages 114–115). When insufflation endotracheal anaesthesia was currently used it was at first thought[46] that the pressure of the returning gas stream was sufficient to blow any secretions present out of the trachea. Robinson[47] apparently realized that this was not trustworthy as a method, for in 1915 he stated that "profuse purulent bronchial secretions" are a contra-indication to endotracheal anaesthesia. Later, when insufflation with a double tube was practised, it was found that the return tube could be used as the catheter for the drainage of secretions by suction.[48] In operations involving the tissue of the lung itself haemorrhage into the bronchi may occur, and blood no less than pus must be removed by aspiration. Nor is the danger of drowning the only objection to the presence of pus in the bronchial tree. It has been found that hitherto healthy portions of the lungs can be infected by pus which has drained into them during or just after operation. For this reason it is more satisfactory to prevent pus from reaching healthy alveoli than to drain it after it has contaminated them. Thus far, as we shall see, this has not always proved practicable. It was to facilitate the passage of the suction catheter through the tube that the angle-piece with a side-tube (see Figure 16 on page 60) was devised. The passage of the catheter is facilitated if it is well lubricated beforehand. When suction is applied within the trachea the anaesthetic vapor is naturally sucked out of the respiratory passages. If a closed system is in use a rapid flow of gases must be instituted during the use of suction in order to replace the gases aspirated.

Whenever a suction catheter is used in the bronchus of the diseased lung during lobectomy or pneumonectomy the anaesthetist should make sure, at the appropriate moment, that the catheter has not by mistake been seized when the surgeon applied his snare to the hilar structures, for its inclusion in the suture line might have disastrous consequences.

THE CONTROL OF SURGICAL PNEUMOTHORAX

When the pleural cavity is opened the lung inside the cavity collapses. This collapse results in respiratory embarrassment and deficient ventilation, which vary as the suddenness with which the collapse occurs. It must not be supposed, however, that the creation of a pneumothorax causes the immediate death of the patient. Many empyemata have been successfully drained without recourse to the use of positive pressure, and spinal analgesia has been successfully used in a large number of intrapleural operations since Shields[49] first suggested the technique in 1935. The experience of the last fifteen years has clearly established the fact that the control of the intrapulmonic pressure from within the trachea is easier, more rational, and more efficient than the complex positive and negative pressure cabinets which were in vogue at the beginning of this century. When the pleural cavity is open, intubation is desirable (see page 29) to control the volume of the lungs, and the administration of the anaesthetic must be performed by some method which enables positive pressure to be applied to the anaesthetic vapor. Of these the absorption technique is the more satisfactory because it enables the application of pressure to be intermittent and synchronized with the phases of the respiratory cycle. For efficiency of management with alternating pressure methods it is essential that there shall be no leakage of gases between the tube and the tracheal walls, and therefore either an inflatable cuff or an efficient pack in the pharynx is essential.

CONTROLLED RESPIRATION

During certain thoracic operations the respiratory movements may inconvenience the surgeon. The evolution of the technique of controlled respiration, described on pages 111–112, has enabled the anaesthetist to minimize this inconvenience. It also permits him to abolish the disturbance to the patient of paradoxical breathing, and to spare him some of the exertion of voluntary respiration when in a position which places him at a mechanical disadvantage.

THE DIFFERENTIAL COLLAPSE OF THE LUNGS

In certain operations it is desirable that the lung undergoing operation be collapsed in order that the surgeon shall have room to work. This applies especially to lobectomy and pneumonectomy, but is sometimes useful in other operations. Oxygen and all the anaesthetic gases are rapidly absorbed from the alveoli,[50] and therefore if a main bronchus is occluded the lung tissue supplied by it will rapidly become atelectatic. This collapse is accelerated by the retraction and manipulation in the surgical field which brings pressure to bear on the lung tissue. Respiration is then carried on by the other lung, and under these conditions the diseased lung is both collapsed and immobile. This state can be procured by means of endobronchial intubation.[51, 52]

Endobronchial Intubation.—A Magill tube about thirty centimetres in length, carrying an inflatable cuff, is passed into the trachea. In the adult man the No. 9 size is appropriate; in a woman one size smaller; in children the size can only be guessed at in relation to the size of the child. The tube should be of such a bore as almost to fill the lumen of the main bronchus, and this is of a slightly smaller diameter than the trachea. The tube is passed down with its curve pointing to the side which is to be intubated, and with its proximal end held over into the opposite corner of the mouth, in order to obtain a certain degree of "lateral thrust." As its end passes into the main bronchus the contact with the carina can usually be felt. If any resistance is encountered the tube should be slightly withdrawn. The cuff is then inflated, and the movements of the chest are carefully watched. Restriction of thoracic movement should be seen over the lung whose bronchus has *not* been intubated. Since the upper lobe bronchus comes off the main trunk very close to the bifurcation—especially on the right side—the upper half of the chest on the sound side should be closely watched to be sure that it moves on respiration. Inflation of the lungs from the bag will often help to confirm these points. Since the cuff when inflated occludes both the lumen of the trachea and that of the opposite bronchus, the diseased lung soon collapses. As it is difficult to be certain of the exact position of the tube when a bronchus is thus intubated "blind," Magill[53] has devised an instrument (Figure 40) which consists of a flexible metal tube resembling a bronchoscope, mounted on the outside of an illuminated stylet, and provided with an inflatable cuff. With this tube it is possible to perform bronchial intubation under direct vision and be certain that the upper lobe bronchus on the sound side has not been occluded by mistake. Recently, however, Magill and Nosworthy[54] have found that visual endo-

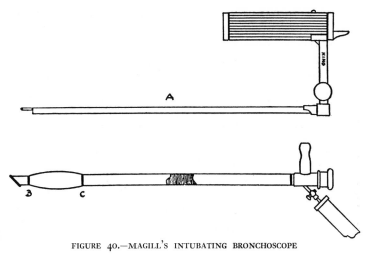

FIGURE 40.—MAGILL'S INTUBATING BRONCHOSCOPE

bronchial intubation can best be performed by placing a bronchoscope of suitable size inside a long Magill tube carrying an inflatable cuff. When intubation has been performed the tube

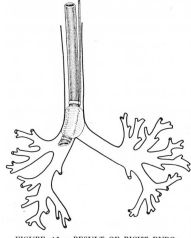

is firmly held in position while the bronchoscope is withdrawn. The result of endobronchial intubation is diagrammatically shown in the figure at the left.

Endobronchial anaesthesia involves the imposition of a considerable strain on the respiratory and circulatory systems by the abrupt inhibition of function of one lung. If the absorptive area of the affected lung has been greatly diminished by the processes of disease, the loss of its surface has probably

FIGURE 41.—RESULT OF RIGHT ENDO-
BRONCHIAL INTUBATION

already been compensated for by the individual; and the disturbance resulting from its collapse is less than it would be had it been functioning normally. When the patient is turned into position for operation, lying on his sound lung, there is often some cyanosis, even if ventilation is manually assured.

THE APPLICATION OF THESE METHODS

We may now examine the application of these principles to the various interventions of thoracic surgery. These fall into three groups: the superficial operations upon the chest wall; the proceedings which involve the opening of the pleural cavity; and the interventions upon the mediastinal structures or upon the substance of the lung itself. Most operations in the first category call for no comment here, since they present none of the special difficulties associated with the other groups. There are two exceptions: the operation of thoracoplasty and the procedures allied to it, and that of extrapleural pneumothorax. These are usually performed as part of the surgical treatment of chronic pulmonary tuberculosis, and therefore the patients may exhibit sputum and require suction drainage of the bronchial tree, and intubation to make this possible. The patient's history is the best guide in determining the necessity for it. Some surgeons perform a bronchoscopic drainage of the respiratory tract immediately before operation, and this sometimes renders further drainage during anaesthesia superfluous. The only other occasion for intubation in these cases is when the anaesthetist finds it impossible either to maintain an accurate apposition of the facepiece or adequate control of the airway in the position of the patient required by the surgeon. The use of controlled respiration may be of assistance in thoracoplasty to prevent paradoxical respiration if the pleural cavity is opened by accident or the integrity of the chest wall is greatly impaired. Thus there are sound arguments in favor of intubation in patients undergoing thoracoplasty. In extrapleural pneumothorax operations drainage is not often necessary, but the establishment of controlled respiration is of assistance to the surgeon. In the position usually used for the operation it is difficult to maintain a sufficiently accurate apposition of the mask to enable inflation to be performed without a constant leakage of gases, and intubation is desirable to overcome this difficulty.

The commonest operation in the second group is that for the drainage of an empyema. The pleural cavity is opened in the course of this intervention, and therefore a pneumothorax is created; but the operation can be rapidly performed, the opening in the pleura is small, and usually adhesions prevent the collapse of the lung. Notwithstanding the fact that Silk[55] in 1918 suggested that intubation was of value in cases of chronic empyema, so many of these operations have been successfully performed without it that we may justifiably assume it to be superfluous. The anaesthetist should, however, be prepared to maintain some degree of positive pressure with the facepiece so that the lung may be prevented from collapsing suddenly when the pleural cavity is first opened; and he should be prepared to intubate at any time should this become necessary.

The other operations in this group are chiefly those in which the trans-pleural route of approach to structures other than the lungs is used. In the majority of these suction is not required. Positive pressure, however, is necessary; and controlled respiration facilitates the performance of the operation. In certain rare cases endobronchial anaesthesia and the complete collapse of the lung on the side of the operation may be desirable in order to facilitate approach. The various operations upon the heart or pericardium, interventions upon the oesophagus or the cardiac end of the stomach by the transthoracic route, the repair of diaphragmatic herniae, or the removal of tumors from the mediastinum can usually be performed efficiently when there is control of the intrapulmonic pressure or controlled respiration has been instituted. The control of pressure consists of the application, just as the pleural cavity is about to be opened, of sufficient positive pressure to hold the lung fully distended. A pressure of six millimetres of mercury is usually sufficient for this purpose, but this varies in every individual. The anaesthetist must watch the degree of distension of the lung and find by direct experiment the minimum pressure which will achieve the desired result in a given patient. Controlled respiration is then maintained during the time that the chest is open. As the last sutures are being inserted for the closure of the pleural cavity the pressure in the breathing bag is raised to the extent necessary just to bring the periphery of the lung up to the level of the pleura during the inspiratory phase. This pressure is maintained until the suture line is tied. In the case of the closed system of maintenance this is achieved by manual pressure on the bag: if the semiclosed system is in use the expiratory valve is tightened so that the pressure in the bag rises to the necessary extent. In these cases, therefore, intubation is of value. The dangers inherent in the use of excessive positive pressure have already been discussed on pages 112–115. No more pressure should ever be used than is necessary to achieve the purpose.

There remain for consideration the three operations undertaken upon the substance of the lung itself. Each of these presents its own specific problems.

The Drainage of a Pulmonary Abscess.—Fortunately abscesses usually occur in a lower lobe, which is the easier of the two for the anaesthetist to isolate from the remainder of the respiratory tract. Moreover, operative interference is usually not undertaken until adhesions have formed between the lung and the pleura. The problems associated with pneumothorax are therefore to some extent avoided. The chief danger arises from the fact that pus and blood are often liberated into the bronchi in a constant trickle. Drainage of the bronchial tree by suction is therefore essential; and it may be carried out either by the passage of a small coudé catheter outside the endotracheal tube, as recommended by Magill and quoted by Hewer,[56] or by means of a catheter passed through the endotracheal tube. Such an arrangement has three drawbacks:

1. Pus accidentally liberated from the abscess may not be removed rapidly enough by the suction, and some may find its way into the unaffected lobes.

2. When a pulmonary abscess is opened a broncho-pleural fistula often results, and the anaesthetic gases then escape into the air through this opening. Air may also enter through the fistula and upset the smoothness of the anaesthesia by dilution of the gases.

3. The lungs cannot be inflated, partly because the constant trickle of blood and pus down the bronchus from the site of operation demands almost continuous suction, and partly because inflation merely drives the vapor into the outside air through the fistula. The suction naturally removes much of the anaesthetic atmosphere, which must be constantly replenished by a rapid flow of gases into the tube. Waters (see page 44) has pointed out that this condition resembles the insufflation of Meltzer and Auer (see page 36) with the direction of flow of the gases reversed. They are blown in through the endotracheal tube and sucked out by the catheter. In practice, however, it is found that a fair degree of ventilation can be obtained by this method even if the respiratory movements are minimal or absent.

Probably the ideal solution in this type of operation would be the technique suggested by Magill[53] for lower lobectomy: a small suction catheter carrying an inflatable cuff inserted be-

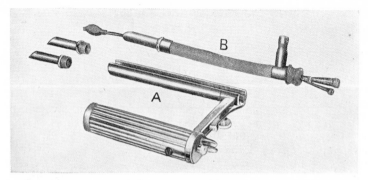

FIGURE 42.—MAGILL'S TRACHEOSCOPE (A) AND SUCTION TUBE (B)

low the upper lobe bronchus by means of a tracheoscope
(Figure 42) and anaesthesia administered by means of the tube
of the tracheoscope. This method, whose results are shown
diagrammatically in Figure 43, isolates the diseased lobe without
interfering with respiration in the healthy portions of the lungs.
As an alternative, endobronchial anaesthesia of the sound lung
may be administered, while the secretions are removed by means
of a catheter in the bronchus of the diseased lung.

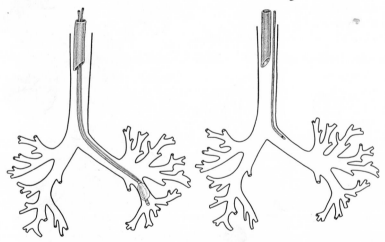

FIGURE 43.—RESULTS OF THE USE   FIGURE 44.—MAGILL'S ORIGINAL METHOD
OF MAGILL'S TRACHEOSCOPE   OF BRONCHIAL SUCTION DRAINAGE

Lobectomy.—An ideal method of anaesthesia for the operation of lobectomy has yet to be discovered. In 1930 Magill[57] felt that intubation was superfluous. Within the next five years, however, he suggested the passage of a small coudé suction catheter just into the bronchus of the affected side while anaesthesia was maintained by means of an endotracheal tube. This arrangement is shown diagrammatically in Figure 44. It was found, however, that this technique did nothing to prevent infection of the remaining lobe from secretions aspirated into it. In 1936 Magill[53] proposed the use of the tracheoscope armed with a long cuffed suction catheter (Figure 42) and the technique illustrated in Figure 43. This seems ideal in theory, but reports on its use are not as yet numerous enough to justify any statement as to its value in practice. As yet, however, no solution has been forthcoming to the problem of how to achieve a similar result in the case of upper lobectomies. Endobronchial anaesthesia may be employed, but while it offers the surgeon the advantage of a collapsed lung upon which to operate and protects the sound lung from infection, it does not protect the remaining lobe on the side of the operation. If endobronchial anaesthesia is used in lobectomy the remaining lobe should be re-inflated at the close of the operation and after all secretions have been aspirated, by withdrawing the tube from the bronchus, re-inflating the cuff, and exerting gentle manual pressure on the bag. Rovenstine[52] recommends the use of a tube carrying two cuffs for this purpose, so that the inflation can be achieved by deflating the endobronchial cuff and inflating the endotracheal cuff without moving the tube.

Pneumonectomy.—Endobronchial anaesthesia is well adapted to the operation of pneumonectomy. The technique of intubation has been described on pages 154–156. Since the diseased lung is entirely removed at operation the question of residual intrapulmonary infection does not arise. The operating conditions are excellent, and the sound lung is protected from the aspiration of foreign fluids or fragments of tissue accidentally broken off.

It will be evident from the foregoing that in anaesthesia for

thoracic operations the use of an inflatable cuff is usually desirable, and that, to facilitate suction and ensure an adequate
airway, tubes of adequate calibre should be used. There are no
cogent reasons for nasotracheal intubation in thoracic cases.
Since narrower tubes must be used through the nose, and the
course of the tube is more curved (see Figure 28 on page 87)
the passage of a suction catheter is more difficult through a
nasal than through an oral tube. Hence there is general agreement with the view expressed by Magill[58] and Rovenstine[52]
that nasal intubation should not be used in anaesthesia for
thoracic operations.

In 1939 Dunlop[59] published an epitome of numerous replies
to a questionnaire soliciting workers' views on anaesthesia for
thoracic operations. The wide divergences of opinion revealed
suggest that we do not yet possess enough experience in the
management of these cases to evaluate the merits of any method
dogmatically. The intubation of these patients, however, is of
sufficient technical difficulty to warrant the supposition that the
trauma inflicted by the inexpert has created an undue prejudice
against the use of endotracheal anaesthesia in thoracic cases.

IN ABDOMINAL OPERATIONS

As we have seen (see pages 26–27), it has been recognized
since 1903 that endotracheal anaesthesia, by overcoming spasm
of the glottis, ensures the ability to procure that smooth and
deep anaesthesia which is desirable, if not essential, in abdominal
interventions. The following reasons for this seem pertinent.
First: when the glottis is open, "straining" no longer raises the
intra-abdominal pressure efficiently. When the recti abdominis
contract the diaphragm rises and the lungs are compressed. This
is why patients who have undergone laryngectomy find it difficult to strain at stool, and why women in labor cannot "bear
down" unless they hold their breath at the same time. Secondly:
if the glottis does not close reflexly in response to surgical stimulus, there is no interference with the freedom of airway necessary for the establishment of deep anaesthesia. Moreover, the
anaesthetist can nullify by manual ventilation the lack of oxygen
and excess of carbon dioxide to which closure of the glottis

otherwise gives rise. Since both these conditions give rise to an artificial muscular rigidity, better relaxation can be obtained by intubation. These advantages can be equally well achieved by the production of a plane of anaesthesia sufficiently deep to cause a complete paralysis of the vocal cords. Provided the anaesthetist is prepared to do this, and is sufficiently skilful to ensure the absolute freedom of airway necessary, intubation becomes superfluous in abdominal operations. A number of anaesthetists feel that lighter anaesthesia, and an intubation which enables them to secure adequate relaxation in this state, involves less strain on the patient than the maintenance of a plane of anaesthesia sufficiently deep to cause abolition of the glottic reflex. The modern tendency is to use lighter anaesthesia and intubation. Opinions differ as to whether this is a wiser course than to practise deeper anaesthesia without intubation. Dawkins[60] and Hornabrook[61] feel that the modern habit of intubating before lower abdominal operations is a mistake. Without doubt intubation has often been practised without reasonable cause, especially in recent years. The present state of our knowledge does not enable us to adjudicate between these two schools of thought; the question will be settled only by the future testimony of accurately kept records of many cases anaesthetized by both methods under comparable conditions.

Nevertheless intubation has certain further advantages in particular abdominal cases that must not be overlooked. It should be resorted to for any operation in the course of which vomiting—whether the active vomiting of a recent meal or the passive regurgitation of "faecal vomiting"—may occur. This applies to all cases of acute intestinal obstruction from whatever cause, and to any patient who is known to have ingested a meal shortly before operation. In these patients an inflatable cuff on the endotracheal tube is an absolute safeguard against the aspiration of vomitus when once the tube is in place and the cuff inflated. This advantage of endotracheal anaesthesia is accepted without debate by most workers.[62]

Many gastric surgeons now feel that it is an advantage if a stomach tube can be passed during the operation. Unless intubation is practised this cannot be done without interrupting the administration and therefore the smoothness of the anaesthetic. Whenever the nature of an abdominal operation makes it desirable to maintain controlled respiration (see page 111) in order to provide a motionless field of work for the surgeon, intubation with an inflatable cuff is the ideal technique. This is not essential, but if an "open" intubation is used and the mask is replaced on the face, it may often happen that the manual pressure on the bag forces the vapor not only into the lungs but also into the stomach. There results a large distended stomach which is a hindrance to the surgeon and may necessitate the passage of a stomach tube for its relief. If, on the other hand, an "open" intubation is performed and the tube is then connected to the breathing bag, much of the anaesthetic vapor is lost by leakage between the cords and the tube with each compression of the breathing bag. This leads to sudden variations in the level of anaesthesia.

Almost all abdominal cases can be quite satisfactorily anaesthetized without intubation; the more skilful the anaesthetist the more rarely will he be forced to resort to intubation. Difficulties encountered during induction often justify a premonition that severe glottic spasm will ensue on surgical stimulus. In such cases it is probably wise to intubate forthwith as an insurance against future troubles.

The author[63] recently made the statement that "glottic spasm is unpredictable in its behaviour and dangerous inasmuch as the anaesthetist cannot control it. Therefore it should be made impossible as early in the course of anaesthesia as is practicable." A communication[64] in the *British Journal of Anaesthesia* well illustrates this point, for it reports four cases of severe spasm of the glottis, two of which ended fatally within twenty-four hours. These could have been prevented had intubation been resorted to as prophylaxis rather than as treatment.

IN OPERATIONS IN DIFFICULT POSITIONS

When the performance of the operation makes it necessary for the patient to be placed in a position in which either his respiratory movements are mechanically hindered or the anaesthetist cannot effectively control the airway or the fit of the facepiece, the advisability of endotracheal anaesthesia should be considered. The more skilful and experienced the anaesthetist, the less frequently will he be compelled to intubate. Nothing but a wide experience of similar cases both with and without intubation can teach any individual worker the arguments in its favor. It is sometimes said that endotracheal anaesthesia is a "lazy way of giving an anaesthetic." This is true only where the anaesthetist is a technician pure and simple, who has no other contribution to make to the conduct of the operation. If, however, it is his function to assume the responsibility for the integrity of the patient's circulatory and respiratory systems during operation, he will have little opportunity for indolence during maintenance. Indeed, the greater freedom from preoccupation with the purely mechanical details of the administration enables him to pay closer attention to the patient's condition. In the author's view intubation should always be considered when the operation is to be performed with the patient in the prone position; for in this position not only is respiratory movement much embarrassed, but it is difficult to ensure an adequate apposition of the mask. Intubation is especially important in those orthopaedic operations which are performed in a "plaster bed," since here the control of the airway may be difficult if not impossible. Reductions of fractures of the vertebrae are sometimes performed in positions involving the suspension of the patient by the legs in the prone position, with the chest resting on the table, and in these cases intubation may be the one practical solution to otherwise insuperable mechanical difficulties.

Finally, where an emergency arises which necessitates the maintenance of anaesthesia by a person untrained in the subject, a preliminary intubation by his supervisor may convert a constant source of worry and danger into a safe and smooth administration.

REFERENCES

1. ELSBERG, C. A. Ann. Surg. 1911. LIII. 749.
2. WOOLSEY, W. C. N. Y. State Jour. Med. 1912. XII. 167.
3. MENNELL, Z. Proc. Roy. Soc. Med. (Anaes.) 1922. XV. 13.

4. ———Brit. Jour. Anaes. 1930. VII. 52.
5. BROWN, G.   Med. Jour. Aus. 1931. I. 258.
6. ———Curr. Res. Anaes. & Analg. 1932. XI. 94.
7. BROWN, W. E.   Curr. Res. Anaes. & Analg. 1924. III. 123.
8. LUNDY, J. S. and TUOHY, E. B.   Proc. Staff Meetings Mayo Clinic, 1937. XII. 225.
9. CHALLIS, J. H. T.   Proc. Roy. Soc. Med. (Anaes.) 1933. XXVI. 957.
10. McKESSON, E. I., McCARTHY, K. C., and CLEMENT, F. W.   Curr. Res. Anaes. & Analg. 1934. XIII. 95.
11. GILLESPIE, N. A.   Endotracheal Nitrous Oxide-Oxygen-Ether Anaesthesia in Neurological Surgery. 1934. Unpublished Thesis. Bodleian Library, Oxford.
12. ———Curr. Res. Anaes. & Analg. 1935. XIV. 225.
13. BRENNAN, H. J.   Lancet, 1938. I. 315.
14. LUNDY, J. S. and TOVELL, R. M.   Proc. Staff Meetings Mayo Clinic, 1935. X. 257.
15. JONES, O. M. G.   Personal Communication. 1934.
16. KILNER, T. P.   St. Thomas' Hosp. Repts. 1937. II. 127.
17. BALLANCE, C. and DUEL, A. B.   Arch. Otolaryngol. 1932. XV. 1.
18. MORRIS, W. M.   Lancet, 1938. I. 429.
19. CLEMENT, F. W. and McCARTHY, K. C.   Curr. Res. Anaes. & Analg. 1937. XVI. 101.
20. McCARTHY, K. C.   Anaesthesiology, 1940. I. 216.
21. CHALLIS, J. H. T.   Curr. Res. Anaes. & Analg. 1937. XVI. 82.
22. HEWER, C. L.   Recent Advances in Anaesthesia & Analgesia. 3d ed. Philadelphia, 1939. pp. 233-235.
23. SOUTTAR, H. S.   Brit. Med. Jour. 1934. II. 797.
24. ———Brit. Med. Jour. 1935. II. 777.
25. MAGILL, I. W.   Am. Jour. Surg. 1936. XXXIV. 450.
26. NESBIT, W. M. and WATERS, R. M.   Unpublished Data.
27. MAGILL, I. W.   Proc. Roy. Soc. Med. (Anaes.) 1927. XX. 1301.
28. CHRISTIANSEN, G. W. and McCARTHY, K. C.   Curr. Res. Anaes. & Analg. 1940. XIX. 211.
29. FLOREN.   Therap. Monatsh. 1902. XVI. 507.
30. KELLY, R. E.   Brit. Med. Jour. 1937. II. 678.
31. JOLL, C. A.   Brit. Med. Jour. 1937. II. 679.
32. DUNHILL, T. P.   Proc. Roy. Soc. Med. (Anaes.) 1927. XXI. 345.
33. HEWER, C. L. and KEYNES, G.   Brit. Med. Jour. 1937. II. 724.
34. LEWIS, I. N.   Brit. Med. Jour. 1937. II. 630.
35. WATERS, R. M. Trans. Am. Soc. Anaes. Dec. 8, 1938. p. 15.
36. LAHEY, F. H.   New England Jour. Med. 1939. CCXXI. 978.
37. PETERSON, M. C. and ROVENSTINE, E. A.   Curr. Res. Anaes. & Analg. 1936. XV. 300.
38. MAGILL, I. W. and CLAUSEN, R. J.   (In discussion) Proc. Roy. Soc. Med. (Anaes.) 1925. XIX. 8.
39. TUCKER, G.   J. A. M. A. 1932. XCIX. 1899.
40. GILLESPIE, N. A.   Brit. Jour. Anaes. 1939. XVII. 2.
41. KAYE, G.   Aus. and N-Z Jour. Surg. 1937. VII. 136.
42. EDWARDS, A. T.   Personal Communication. 1938.

43. AYRE, P. Brit. Jour. Surg. 1937. XXV. 131.
44. ————Curr. Res. Anaes. & Analg. 1937. XVI. 330.
45. LEIGH, M. D. and FITZGERALD, R. R. C. M. A. J. 1936. XXXV. 427.
46. MELTZER, S. J. Medical Record, 1910. LXXVII. 477.
47. ROBINSON, S. Surg. Gyn. & Obs. 1915. XXI. 774.
48. MACKENZIE, J. R. Brit. Jour. Anaes. 1932. X. 19.
49. SHIELDS, H. J. Curr. Res. Anaes. & Analg. 1935. XIV. 193.
50. CORYLLOS, P. N. and BIRNBAUM, G. L. Am. Jour. Med. Sci. 1932. CLXXXIII. 326.
51. GALE, J. W. and WATERS, R. M. Jour. Thor. Surg. 1932. I. 432.
52. ROVENSTINE, E. A. Surg. Gyn. & Obs. 1936. LXIII. 325.
53. MAGILL, I. W. Brit. Jour. Anaes. 1936. XIII. 92.
54. MAGILL, I. W. and NOSWORTHY, M. D. Personal Communications. 1941.
55. SILK, F. W. Proc. Roy. Soc. Med. (Anaes.) 1918. XI. 3.
56. HEWER, C. L. Curr. Res. Anaes. & Analg. 1935. XIV. 120.
57. MAGILL, I. W. Proc. Roy. Soc. Med. (Anaes.) 1930. XXIII. 778.
58. ————Personal Communication. 1940.
59. DUNLOP, J. G. Curr. Res. Anaes. & Analg. 1939. XVIII. 301.
60. DAWKINS, C. J. M. Brit. Jour. Anaes. 1937. XIV. 45.
61. HORNABROOK, F. W. Curr. Res. Anaes. & Analg. 1931. X. 248.
62. STAFF OF THE ALFRED HOSP. MELBOURNE. Practical Anaesthetics. 1932. p. 148.
63. GILLESPIE, N. A. Anaesthesiology, 1940. I. 292.
64. Anonymous Correspondence. Brit. Jour. Anaes. 1938. XV. 130.

IX. THE USES OF INTUBATION FOR PURPOSES OTHER THAN ANAESTHESIA

RESUSCITATION

It has already been pointed out on page 6 that intubation as a resuscitative measure was known and practised for several centuries before the discovery of anaesthesia. An extensive and interesting literature on the subject well repays a detailed investigation, which is, however, beyond the scope of the present work. The historical papers by Cotton and Boothby[1] in 1913 and by Waters *et al.*[2] in 1933 make a good introduction to the subject for those interested in pursuing it. The former paper contains a bibliography which is probably complete up to the date of its publication.

In a number of the emergencies of normal life intubation is of value because of the freedom of airway it assures. The resuscitation of persons apparently drowned is facilitated by it, and it was extensively used for this purpose in Paris in the eighteenth and nineteenth centuries.[3] When a person has succumbed to the effects of poisonous or asphyxiant gases, intubation of the trachea is a valuable aid to the application of effective artificial respiration. Of recent years Flagg[4] has drawn attention to its importance, and has organized a society whose function it is to make the means of effective resuscitation known and available.

Intubation is equally valuable in the medical emergencies arising from respiratory arrest or depression. The work of O'Dwyer on intubation in diphtheria (page 9) showed that if the arrest is of obstructive origin, intubation will relieve it as effectively as tracheotomy. If respiration has ceased or is very feeble laryngoscopy must be resorted to, since there are no audible breath sounds to enable blind intubation to be performed. Moreover, time is of the utmost importance, and visual intubation can be accomplished immediately and with certainty. If the obstruction is in the trachea, intubation is usually easy; but intubation for the relief of obstruction caused by an acute infection in the pharynx presents grave difficulties. Often so much oedema of all the structures is present that laryngoscopy is impossible. There is usually some respiratory exchange in these patients; and if so, skill in blind intubation may well save a life.

Respiratory arrest or depression may occur because of a failure of function of the respiratory centre. This may be due to the processes of disease, such as an increase in intracranial pressure resulting from a cerebral abscess or neoplasm; or to an overdose of some drug which depresses the respiratory centre, such as opium or the barbituric acid derivatives. Or arrest or depression may result from lesions of the spinal nerves, either following acute anterior poliomyelitis or trauma causing a paralysis of the muscles of respiration. In all these conditions the ability to maintain adequate gaseous exchange holds out the only hope of saving the patient. The patency of the airway assured by intubation enhances the value of any method of artificial respiration. Fortunately in these patients the structures are usually in a state of utter flaccidity which makes laryngoscopy and intubation easy.

There is no evidence to suggest a limit to the time during which a tube can be left in position in the trachea. When patients succumb to the effects of respiratory dysfunction and an autopsy is performed, lesions for which the tube is held responsible are often found in the respiratory passages. On the other hand, when the patient recovers he rarely complains of any symptom of damage caused by the intubation. In any event all these conditions represent so imminent a danger to life that the possibility of trauma from the intubation becomes a secondary consideration. A tube in the trachea, however, interferes with the processes of deglutition and causes the patient more discomfort than does a tracheotomy tube. If, therefore, the circumstances are such that the tube must remain in place for a long time, it is wiser to perform tracheotomy at once. This must always be done if for some reason intubation does not succeed.

In certain cases of trauma resulting in haemorrhage into the upper air passages intubation may prove to be a life-saving measure. It will ensure a free airway while temporary haemostasis is secured by means of packing, until deliberate ligation of the vessels can be undertaken. This use of intubation is important under conditions of modern warfare.

Not only endoscopists and anaesthetists but all medical men should be sufficiently familiar with the technique of laryngoscopy to be able to exploit the advantages accruing to intubation in such cases without delay. If intubation involves delay, then it hinders rather than helps resuscitation; for it is only the means to the end of restoring efficient respiratory exchange at the earliest possible moment.

IN ASPHYXIA NEONATORUM

No less than in other varieties of asphyxia is intubation valuable as an aid to resuscitation in the new-born infant. Here again the method is of considerable antiquity, having been in use for at least a century. In recent years it has been advocated by De Lee,[5] Flagg,[6] Gibberd and Blaikley,[7,8] and Nosworthy.[9] De Lee practises and recommends tactile intubation, whereas Flagg and Gibberd and Blaikley prefer the visual method, and Nosworthy describes both. Owing to the flaccidity of the asphyxiated infant all the difficulties encountered in intubating normal infants disappear. There is no need even to elevate the epiglottis with the laryngoscope, for if the root of the tongue is lifted it pulls the other structures forwards after it, and the entire hypopharynx lies exposed to view.[7] Under these circumstances intubation is very easy.

A due sense of proportion developed by long clinical experience is required for the sound application of this technique. In the great majority of infants intubation is superfluous, and all that is required is the efficient removal of foreign substances from the pharynx. If intubation is performed in the normal infant the reflex breath-holding resulting from the irritation of the tube may give rise to a more serious lack of oxygen than the minor degree of obstruction which it was intended to relieve. Intubation should therefore be reserved for the treatment of those cases in which a definite impairment of respiratory function is evident, and should be resorted to as soon as this condition is recognized.

The smallest size of Magill tube is passed (see Table I on page 50) and through it gentle inflation of the lungs with oxygen, or the drainage of fluid by aspiration through an even smaller catheter, may be performed. Suction should never be applied to the endotracheal tube itself, for atelectasis may result (pages 114–115). The endotracheal tube is withdrawn as soon as oxygenation is adequate and spontaneous respiration normal.

"TRACHEO-BRONCHIAL TOILET"

Formerly the terms "ether pneumonia" and "postoperative pneumonia" were used to describe a complication deemed to be almost as inexorable as an Act of God. Of recent years the view has become established that in many cases atelectasis precedes the pneumonia,[10] and that if the collapse is recognized and treated in time pneumonia can be prevented. It is thought that a plug of mucus occludes a small bronchus. The pulmonary tissue supplied by that bronchus soon collapses because the gases contained in its alveoli are absorbed. Infection then rapidly sets in and soon a frank broncho-pneumonia is established[11] unless drainage of the affected portion of the lung is performed. In 1933 Negus[12] pointed out that the drainage of such an area of the lung by bronchoscopic suction was of value. The technique of "tracheo-bronchial toilet" is similar, though simpler, and has yielded satisfactory results at the Wisconsin General Hospital since 1935.[13]* It is performed upon the conscious patient in bed. Effective local analgesia of the nares, pharynx, and glottis is first obtained by spraying these parts during inspiration with a nebulizer containing one of the analgesic solutions in common use (see page 63). Blind nasal intubation is then performed if possible, because it causes less discomfort to the conscious

---

* As has been pointed out on page 18, in 1912 Kühn suggested the drainage of secretions by suction through a small tube passed into the trachea through his wide-bore tube. "Tracheo-bronchial toilet" is merely a new term used to distinguish between this simpler and older manoeuvre and bronchoscopy.

patient than laryngoscopy. This at first seems both formidable and inhuman; yet the majority of patients co-operate willingly if the exact procedure and the reason for it are explained to them beforehand; and their own expressions of the relief which they feel afterwards are sufficient to dispel this view. If blind intubation fails, laryngoscopy is gently performed and the tube is inserted by direct vision. When the tube is in place the spray is directed into it once during inspiration to minimize the intensity of the irritation to which its presence gives rise. A small rubber catheter, well lubricated with vaseline, is passed into the trachea through the tube, and suction is applied to the catheter, which is moved up and down while the head is turned to either side in an effort to cause the catheter to pass well down both main bronchi in turn. The patient's position should be changed during this process in order to promote drainage of the secretions. Violent coughing usually results, and in the majority of cases the character of the patient's pulse rate, his temperature and respiration rate, and the augmentation of the respiratory movements, as well as the radiological findings in the thorax, have shown that re-expansion of the affected area of the lung has taken place.

Mousel[14] and Eversole[10] are of the opinion that in such cases bronchoscopy should be resorted to at once. No doubt there are occasions on which this succeeds where tracheo-bronchial toilet fails. Yet bronchoscopy is a more serious undertaking, demanding greater skill, training, and experience for its atraumatic performance. In less skilled hands tracheo-bronchial toilet is potentially less traumatic. It therefore seems logical to apply the simpler proceeding first, and to have recourse to the more difficult only if the simpler fails.

The drainage of secretions from the trachea by suction has proved of value in types of cases other than the treatment of atelectasis. As Nosworthy[15] has recently pointed out, many patients who are too debilitated to be able to expel their own bronchial secretions by coughing must suffer the effects of respiratory obstruction unless their secretions are removed mechanically. This condition is often seen after thoracic or cerebral operations, or when vomitus has been aspirated into the lungs; and its prompt treatment, either by bronchoscopy or tracheo-bronchial toilet, greatly benefits the patient. The success of this treatment depends upon the promptitude with which the condition is recognized and the expedition with which the treatment is applied. Too often the patient is in extremis before drainage is instituted. Even when they have previously been removed, secretions tend to accumulate again, and therefore aspiration should be repeated as often as may be necessary to ensure freedom of respiration.

THE INSTILLATION OF LIPIODOL

The use of opaque liquids injected into the bronchial tree for purposes of radiological examination has greatly increased. Various techniques have been suggested for the purpose. In 1934 Soulas[16] published his account of a method whereby, after local analgesia of the pharynx and larynx, intubation of the trachea was performed and lipiodol was allowed to run into the bronchi through the tube. Although successful, this was unpleasant to the patient and had certain drawbacks. As the patients are usually children it is not easy to obtain their co-operation in an unpleasant proceeding whose necessity is not apparent to them. Soulas records some cases of collapse, and remarks that certain patients exhibited a severe attack of "suffocating cough."

More recently Lyons[17] has described a technique for this purpose whereby the patient receives a basal narcosis with avertin followed by nitrous oxide–oxygen anaesthesia and nasal intubation, local analgesia of the respiratory tract having first been produced. By passing a rubber catheter through the endotracheal tube the lipiodol can be directed into one or the other main bronchus, and much of it can be removed again by the use of suction after the radiographs have been taken, before the endotracheal tube is taken out. As the nitrous oxide is administered by the carbon dioxide absorption technique, respiratory movements can be temporarily inhibited by controlled respiration (see page 111) so as to facilitate the exposure of the film. This method appears to solve most of the difficulties hitherto associated with this proceeding. Its use in England has recently been reported by Baker.[18] He, however, prefers oro-tracheal intubation for the purpose.

REFERENCES

1. COTTON, F. J. and BOOTHBY, W. M.   Ann. Surg. 1913. LVII. 43.
2. WATERS, R. M., ROVENSTINE, E. A., and GUEDEL, A. E.   Curr. Res. Anaes. & Analg. 1933. XII. 196.
3. MAGENDIE, J.   Jour. de Physiol. 1829. IX. 97.
4. FLAGG, P. J.   Am. Jour. Surg. 1939. XLIV. 373.
5. DE LEE, J. B.   Principles and Practice of Obstetrics. 7th ed. Phila-delphia, 1938. pp. 913-919.
6. FLAGG, P. J.   J. A. M. A. 1928. XCI. 788.
7. GIBBERD, G. F. and BLAIKLEY, J. B.   Lancet, 1935. I. 736.
8. ————Lancet, 1935. II. 138.
9. NOSWORTHY, M. D.   St. Thomas' Hosp. Repts. 1939. IV. 134.
10. EVERSOLE, U. H.   Anaesthesiology, 1940. I. 72.
11. WATERS, R. M.   Anaesthesiology, 1940. I. 136.
12. NEGUS, V. E.   Proc. Roy. Soc. Med. (Anaes.) 1933. XXVI. 1127.
13. HATHAWAY, H. R. and LEIGH, M. D.   Trans. Am. Soc. Anaes. 1939. V. 56.
14. MOUSEL, L. H.   J. A. M. A. 1940. CXV. 899.
15. NOSWORTHY, M. D.   Proc. Roy. Soc. Med. (Surg.) 1940. XXXIV. 95.
16. SOULAS, A.   Hôpital, 1934. XXII. 494.
17. LYONS, S.   Curr. Res. Anaes. & Analg. 1939. XVIII. 168.
18. BAKER, A. H. L.   Brit. Jour. Anaes. 1941. XVII. 112.

BIBLIOGRAPHY AND INDEX

BIBLIOGRAPHY

In addition to the works already quoted in the text, the following may be of interest to readers wishing further to pursue the subjects mentioned. Articles are arranged chronologically.

OTHER WORKS OF KÜHN

Verh. des Suddeut. Laryngol. 1906. XIII. 247.
Zentralbl. f. Chirurg. 1906. XXXIII. 241.
Münch. Med. Woch. 1906. LIII. 655 (Vol. 1).

SUMMARY OF KÜHN'S WORK IN ENGLISH

HAZELHURST, F. Laryngoscope, 1913. XXIII. 1091.

INSUFFLATION: WORKS OF GENERAL INTEREST

ELSBERG, C. A. Berl. Klin. Woch. 1910. XLVII. 957.
LILIENTHAL, H. and ELSBERG, C. A. Berl. Klin. Woch. 1910. XLVII. 958.
MELTZER, S. J. Berl. Klin. Woch. 1910. XLVII. 566.
LILIENTHAL, H. Ann. Surg. 1910. LII. 30.
FISCHER, H. Surg. Gyn. & Obs. 1911. XIII. 566.
QUINBY, W. C. Boston Med. & Surg. Jour. 1911. CLXV. 592.
MELTZER, S. J. Trans. Amer. Surg. Assoc. 1911. XXIX. 217.
KEEN, M. Rapport IIIe. Congres Internat. Soc. de Chir. Bruxelles, 1911. p. 674.
GITHENS, T. and MELTZER, S. J. Proc. Soc. Exp. Biol. & Med. 1912. X. 27.
EHRENFRIED, A. Brit. Med. Jour. 1912. II. 616.
MÜLLER, G. P. International Clinics (Phil.), 1912. II. 175.
LEIGHTON, W. E. Jour. Miss. State Med. Assoc. 1912–13. IX. 79.
SINGLETON, A. O. Texas State Jour. Med. 1912–13. IX. 181.
KRUSKAL, I. D. Surg. Gyn. & Obs. 1913. XVII. 117.
BOYLE, H. E. G. and GASK, G. Proc. Roy. Soc. Med. (Anaes.) 1913. VI. 8.
SHIPWAY, F. E. Proc. Roy. Soc. Med. (Anaes.) 1913. VI. 11.
LAUTENSCHLÄGER, A. Berl. Klin. Woch. 1913. LX. 2093.
FABIAN, J. J. Jour. Mich. State Med. Soc. 1913. XII. 193.
CRAWFORD, H. de L. Dublin Jour. Med. Sci. 1913. CXXXV. 413.
KELLY, R. E. Brit. Jour. Surg. 1913. I. 90.
SHIPWAY, F. E. Brit. Jour. Surg. 1913. I. 101.
BOYLE, H. E. G. Proc. Roy. Soc. Med. (Anaes.) 1914. VII. 28.
NAGLE, F. W. Am. Jour. Surg. (Anaes. Supp.) 1914. XXVIII. 17.
THOMPSON, H. T. and STRUTHERS, J. W. Edin. Med. Jour. 1914. XIII. 146.
JONES, R. L. Lancet, 1914. II. 1087.
KELLY, R. E. Proc. Roy. Soc. Med. (Anaes.) 1914. VII. 25.
BOYLE, H. E. G. Proc. Roy. Soc. Med. (Anaes.) 1914. VII. 28.
WILLIAMS, A. W. J. A. M. A. 1915. LXIV. 138.

RICKETTS, B. M.   Am. Jour. Surg. (Anaes. Supp.) 1915. XXIX. 147.
BILANCIONI, C.   Policlinico, 1917. XXIV. 182.
SHIPWAY, F. E.   Proc. Roy. Soc. Med. (Anaes.) 1920. XIII. 1.
————Am. Jour. Surg. (Anaes. Supp.) 1921. XXXV. 16.
HEPBURN, W. G.   Curr. Res. Anaes. & Analg. 1922. I. 83.
MAGILL, I. W.   Lancet, 1923. II. 68.
KAVANAGH, M.   Am. Jour. Surg. (Anaes. Supp.) 1923. XXXVII. 44.
WEAVER, R. E.   Med. Jour. Aus. 1924. I. 506.
MAGILL, I. W.   Lancet, 1926. I. 461.
STEWART, C. C.   C. M. A. J. 1927. XVII. 1182.
GREEN, F. W.   Curr. Res. Anaes. & Analg. 1928. VII. 201.
WATKINS, A. B. K.   Med. Jour. Aus. 1928. I. 237.
BROWN, G.   Curr. Res. Anaes. & Analg. 1931. X. 285.

INSUFFLATION: EXPERIMENTAL

MELTZER, S. J. and AUER, J.   Zentral. f. Physiol. 1909. XXII. 210 and 443.
ELSBERG, C. A.   Ann. Surg. 1910. LII. 23.
CARREL, A.   La Presse Medicale, 1910. XVIII. 9.
————Berl. Klin. Woch. 1910. XLVII. 565.
LENORMANT, C.   Jour. de Chir. 1910. V. 645.
UNGER, E. and BETTMANN, M.   Berl. Klin. Woch. 1910. XLVII. 959.
MELTZER, S. J. and AUER, J.   Jour. Exper. Med. 1911. XIV. 569.
D'AVACK, A.   Policlinico, 1913. XX. 153.
VAN DEN BERGH and WIERSMAN.   Nederl. Tijdsch. v. Geneesk.
    1914. II. 383.
HIRSCHMANN, C.   (Abstract) J. A. M. A. 1926. LXXXVII. 1691.

APPARATUS FOR INSUFFLATION

EHRENFRIED, A.   Boston Med. & Surg. Jour. 1911. CLXV. 594.
————Med. Comm. Mass. Med. Soc. 1911. XXII. 148.
SALZER, M.   J. A. M. A. 1913. LX. 826.
WOOLSEY, W. C.   Long Island Med. Jour. 1913. VII. 24.
EGIDI, G.   Riv. Ospedalia, 1913. III. 551.
SHIPWAY, F. E.   Bristol Med-Chir. Jour. 1913. XXXI. 341.
ROGERS, J.   Ann. Surg. 1913. LVII. 276.
STOCK, S. V. and FRY, J. D.   Bristol Med-Chir. Jour. 1913. XXXI. 344.
GROVES, E. W. H.   Bristol Med-Chir. Jour. 1913. XXXI. 347.
PRATT, J. P.   J. A. M. A. 1914. LXII. 37.
ROEHRIG, K. F.   Colorado Medicine, 1916. XIII. 188.
SHIPWAY, F. E.   Lancet, 1916. II. 236.
ADSON, A. W. and LITTLE, G. C.   J. A. M. A. 1918. LXX. 1746.
ROWBOTHAM, S.   Lancet, 1921. II. 660.
MAGILL, I. W.   Lancet, 1921. I. 918.
————Lancet, 1923. II. 228.
WATKINS, A. B. K.   Med. Jour. Aus. 1926. II. 48.
MAGILL, I. W.   Lancet, 1927. II. 396.
WATKINS, A. B. K.   Med. Jour. Aus. 1929. II. 191.
KAYE, G.   Med. Jour. Aus. 1929. I. 701.

ARTICLES RELATING TO ACCIDENTS OR TRAUMA

UNGER, E. Berl. Klin. Woch. 1910. XLVII. 1748.
COTTON, F. J. and BOOTHBY, W. M. Boston Med. & Surg. Jour. 1912. CLXVI. 486.
EHRLICH, S. D. Medical Record, 1914. LXXVI. 926.
CLAUSEN, R. J. Brit. Med. Jour. 1935. II. 601.
MAGILL, I. W. Brit. Med. Jour. 1935. II. 639.

TRANSITION TECHNIQUES BETWEEN INSUFFLATION AND INHALATION

LONG, W. H. Kentucky Med. Jour. 1922. XX. 707.
ROWBOTHAM, S. Lancet, 1926. II. 583.
FLAGG, P. J. Arch. Otolaryngol. 1927. V. 394.
HARGRAVE, R. C. M. A. J. 1927. XVII. 688.
STEWART, C. C. C. M. A. J. 1929. XXI. 309.
JONES, W. H. Lancet, 1929. I. 330.
LOEWENTHAL, L. S. Curr. Res. Anaes. & Analg. 1930. IX. 207.
DE CAUX, F. P. Curr. Res. Anaes. & Analg. 1930. IX. 254.
KAYE, G. Med. Jour. Aus. 1932. I. 684.

INHALATION: WORKS OF GENERAL INTEREST

DAVIES, H. M. Brit. Med. Jour. 1911. II. 61.
HARGRAVE, R. Brit. Jour. Anaes. 1928. VI. 98.
BROWN, G. Curr. Res. Anaes. & Analg. 1931. X. 285.
AUSTIN, L. T. Coll. Papers Mayo Clinic, 1932. XXIV. 1027.
FULLERTON, F. W. N-Z Med. Jour. 1932. XXXI. 31.
MINNITT, R. J. Liverpool Med. Chir. Jour. 1932. XL. 168.
STEWART, C. C. C. M. A. J. 1933. XXVIII. 295.
SHAW, R. W. Irish Jour. Med. Sci. 1934. 6th Series. p. 654.
TOVELL, R. M. Surg. Clinics of N. America, 1935. XV. 1277.
KAYE, G. Brit. Med. Jour. 1935. II. 618.
MALAN, E. Il Valsalva, 1935. XI. 508.
MONOD, R., AUBIN, A., and THIERRY, F. Anesthésie Analgésie, 1936. II. 422.
AUBIN, A. Anesthésie Analgésie, 1936. II. 590.
FLAGG, P. J. Arch. Otolaryngol. 1937. XXV. 405.
HARGRAVE, R. Curr. Res. Anaes. & Analg. 1937. XVI. 181.
THOMAS, G. J. Curr. Res. Anaes. & Analg. 1938. XVII. 301.
HUMAN, J. U. The Secrets of Blind Intubation and the Signs of Anaesthesia. London, 1938.
CLEMENT, F. W. Nitrous Oxide-Oxygen Anaesthesia. Phil. 1939. pp. 165–176.
CLEMENT, F. W. Jour. Indiana State Med. Assoc. 1940. XXXIII. 13.
GILLIES, H. D. et al. Brit. Med. Jour. 1940. I. 69.
KELLY, R. E. Brit. Med. Jour. 1940. I. 107.
MAGILL, I. W. Brit. Med. Jour. 1940. I. 150.
SHERIDAN, M. R. Brit. Med. Jour. 1940. I. 231.
HEWER, C. L. Brit. Med. Jour. 1940. I. 318.

MODIFIED MAGILL TUBES

MURPHY, F. J.   Curr. Res. Anaes. & Analg. 1941. XX. 102.

LARYNGOSCOPES

ARBUCKLE, M. F.   Curr. Res. Anaes. & Analg. 1940. XIX, Supplement, p. 130.
MILLER, R. A.   Anaesthesiology, 1941. II. 317.

ENDOTRACHEAL ANAESTHESIA IN THORACIC SURGERY

LIDWILL, M.   Curr. Res. Anaes. & Analg. 1926. V. 142.
HEWER, C. L.   Curr. Res. Anaes. & Analg. 1930. IX. 24.
————Brit. Med. Jour. 1930. I. 286.
MAGILL, I. W.   Proc. Roy. Soc. Med. (Anaes.) 1936. XXIX. 643.
EVERSOLE, U. H. and OVERHOLT, R.   Jour. Thor. Surg. 1936. V. 510.
HALTON, J.   Lancet, 1940. II. 675.
BEECHER, H. K.   Jour. Thor. Surg. 1940. X. 202.
PHILLIPS, F., LIVINGSTONE, H. M., and ADAMS, W. E.   Curr. Res. Anaes.
    & Analg. 1941. XX. 78.
NOSWORTHY, M. D.   Proc. Roy. Soc. Med. (Anaes.) 1941. XXXIV. 479.

INDEX